RE

MADRONA

"*Bedlam* moves in gentle and revelatory proximity to people striving to survive one of America's worst public policy mistakes. Dr. Ken Rosenberg's gifts as a reporter and bold storyteller are a godsend to the one in five American families grappling with serious mental illness."

—SALLY JO FIFER, PRESIDENT AND CEO, INDEPENDENT
TELEVISION SERVICE

"*Bedlam* blazes new ground in that it shows all the multifaceted problems faced by the seriously mentally ill using their own words and experiences. It then brilliantly interweaves their narratives with savvy policy prescriptions."

—DJ JAFFE, AUTHOR OF *INSANE CONSEQUENCES* AND EXECUTIVE
DIRECTOR, MENTAL ILLNESS POLICY ORG.

"The United States has become the worst place in the world to have a severe mental illness. Ken Rosenberg describes this American nightmare with the stark vividness of painful firsthand experience—as brother, as psychiatrist, and as visionary documentary filmmaker who explains how we got into this barbaric mess and suggests commonsense, cost-effective ways to regain our societal sanity."

—ALLEN FRANCES, MD, PROFESSOR AND CHAIR EMERITUS, DUKE
DEPARTMENT OF PSYCHIATRY, CHAIR OF DSM-IV TASK FORCE, AND AUTHOR
OF *SAVING NORMAL*

BEDLAM

AN INTIMATE JOURNEY
INTO AMERICA'S
MENTAL HEALTH CRISIS

KENNETH PAUL ROSENBERG, MD

with JESSICA DuLONG

AVERY | AN IMPRINT OF PENGUIN RANDOM HOUSE | NEW YORK

AVERY

An imprint of Penguin Random House LLC
penguinrandomhouse.com

Most Avery books are available at special quantity discounts for bulk purchase for sales promotions, premiums, fund-raising, and educational needs. Special books or book excerpts also can be created to fit specific needs. For details, write SpecialMarkets@ penguinrandomhouse.com.

Library of Congress Cataloging-in-Publication Data

Names: Rosenberg, Kenneth Paul, author. | DuLong, Jessica, author.
Title: Bedlam: an intimate journey into America's mental health crisis /
Kenneth Rosenberg, Jessica DuLong.
Description: New York: Avery, 2019. | Includes bibliographical references and index. |
Identifiers: LCCN 2019021479 | ISBN 9780525541318 (hardcover) |
ISBN 9780525541325 (ebook)
Subjects: LCSH: Mental health services—United States. |
Mental health policy—United States. | Mentally ill—Care—Case studies. |
Mentally ill—United States—Social conditions.
Classification: LCC RA790.6.R662 2019 | DDC 362.20973—dc23
LC record available at https://lccn.loc.gov/2019021479

Printed in the United States of America
1   3   5   7   9   10   8   6   4   2

Book design by Lorie Pagnozzi

For the one in five families

CONTENTS

AUTHOR'S NOTE

I used the real names of most of the people in this project, with their permission. Despite that permission, I changed a few names and identifying details in circumstances where I felt inclusion could be harmful to certain individuals. I also streamlined quotes for clarity.

On the matter of consent: since med school, I have been working to bring documentary stories about mental illness to public and professional attention. As I wrote this book, I made a film for PBS that documents some of the same patients and doctors profiled here. Long before obtaining consents, I spent roughly two years with Los Angeles County + University of Southern California (LAC+USC) Medical Center and Los Angeles County officials to review our protocol for filming patients responsibly. Our agreed-upon procedure was for the emergency department (ED) staff to first ask a patient and authorize consent before the patient was introduced to me or any member of my team. In all cases in which I followed a patient closely, I spoke with them (and whenever possible with their family members) over the course of at least five years, to ask them repeatedly for their permission to tell their stories. This close, long-term follow-up promoted a unique collaboration: rather than a project *about* a glimpse of patients and doctors in the ED over a few hours, the project became a close and ongoing collaboration *with* the doctors, patients, and families to tell their stories as they evolved over the course of time.

Aside from the patients and families, this project also has many collaborators, whom I thank in the acknowledgments. I cannot sufficiently thank my film team, which includes Peter Miller, Bob Richman, Buddy Squires, Jim Cricchi, Enat Sidi, Lynn Novick, and Anthony Simon. Because of the virtuoso and empathic work of my co-producers, Los Angeles cameraperson and director of photography Joan Churchill, and location sound recordist Alan Barker, I was able to record the words and lives of the subjects even when I couldn't be in L.A. Executive Producer of Independent Lens Lois Vossen, Independent Television Service (ITVS) CEO Sally Jo Fifer, and ITVS Supervising Producer Shana Swanson pushed me to tell the story of our country's abandonment of persons with mental illnesses that had never been told fully on television. I am indebted to the John D. and Catherine T. MacArthur Foundation Journalism and Media Program, National Alliance on Mental Illness, the American Psychiatric Association, the Los Angeles Department of Health, the Los Angeles Department of Mental Health, the National Institute of Mental Health, the Substance Abuse and Mental Health Services Administration, JusticeLA, Power and Dignity Now, and the many organizations who've supported me.

This book would not exist but for the combination of the efforts of my agent and guiding light, Joy Tutela; my editor, Nina Shield, at Avery Publishing (an imprint of Penguin Random House), who brilliantly kept me focused on both the big picture and the details; and my close collaborator, Jessica DuLong, who brought her formidable skills as a gifted writer and conscientious journalist to every aspect of this project. Impeccable fact-checking was done by Elizabeth Sinclair and attorney Brian Stettin, both of whom work at the Treatment Advocacy Center as research director and policy director, respectively.

I am most thankful to the patients, families, and health care providers who opened their lives and hearts to us. I hope our work does justice to their generosity and the trust that they placed in our team. Inspired by the bravery of the people whom we profiled, I decided to share my own story in a way that I never thought possible. For that alone, I am immeasurably grateful.

INTRODUCTION

My family's tragedy is an American tragedy. My family's shame is America's great secret. In this country, one in five adults (and one in five families) lives with a mental illness, according to the National Institute of Mental Health (NIMH).[1] Of that total, an estimated 11.2 million people age eighteen or older have a serious mental illness (SMI), leading to some degree of functional impairment.[2]

This book is largely about adults with SMI, but I need to clarify the term. In medical and scientific terms, SMI includes all cases of schizophrenia, disabling mood and thought disorders, severe bipolar disorder, severe depression, and other psychiatric conditions that I will discuss in detail. SMI is also an economic and political designation that helps federal, state, and local agencies distribute grants on behalf of the sickest psychiatric patients. Although it is easy to differentiate people with an SMI from those who have relatively minor problems of living—the so-called worried well—it is more challenging to figure out if SMI includes folks with disabling panic attacks, disruptive personality disorders, and post-traumatic stress disorders (PTSD). Substance abuse disorders and addictive relationships to drugs and alcohol are not officially considered a kind of SMI. But if you ask me, these diseases, which affect more than 15 percent of the population at some point in their lives and can be fatal, also belong in that camp.[3]

The counterpart to SMI among children is serious emotional disturbance (SED), affecting approximately 7 to 12 percent of children.[4] A person age eighteen or under is said to have SED if they currently, or at any time during the past year, have had a diagnosable mental, behavioral, or emotional disorder that "has resulted in functional impairment which substantially interferes with or limits the child's role or functioning in family, school, or community activities."[5] SEDs do not include substance abuse disorders or developmental disorders like mental retardation; they are emotional illnesses like suicidal depression, bipolar disorder, and severe attention deficit disorder (ADD).[6]

Aside from implying a high level of impairment, the terms SMI and SED generally refer to illness for which there is no known biological cause. They are mysterious disruptions in thoughts, emotions, and behavior usually without any identifiable brain damage, as is visible in cases of Alzheimer's disease, a stroke, or advanced HIV disease. In the twentieth century, many psychiatrists thought SMIs were largely due to problems of nurture, like psychological damage inflicted by harsh and inconsistent parents. Today, most think that, unlike less serious disorders, they result from biology, at least to some degree. This binary between organic and psychological diseases is likely to recede as we discover more about the mind and the brain and recognize that our biology and psychology are constantly interacting with each other and influencing our behaviors.

• • •

Any discussion of mental illness begins and ends with the sense of shame surrounding mental illness that is alive and well,[7] often stemming from the perception that people with SMI or their families are to blame, and education alone does not seem capable of reversing the public's misconception. Consider, for example, the way the term *schizophrenic* is used pejoratively, with no relationship to the actual disease. How did people with serious psychiatric disorders feel when an outgoing White House communications director called a White House chief of staff "a fucking paranoid schizophrenic"?[8] "Stigma causes people to feel ashamed for something that *is* out of their control," explains Laura Greenstein of the National Alliance on Mental Illness (NAMI). "Worst of all, stigma prevents people from seeking the help they need." This book is very much about stigma.

From both my family and my work, I have long had a sense of how terrible things are for individuals with SMI and their loved ones. Yet until I set out on my quest for understanding how my family's struggles fit into the struggles of the nation as a whole, I did not fully appreciate the degree to which our country has come to abandon our sickest citizens—or what we might do to change things.

I failed to appreciate our *criminalization* of people with mental illness, which refers to putting them in jails and prisons instead of into institutions of healing. I've learned that our criminalization goes much deeper—allowing sick people to languish in the streets, calling the police to pick them up when they become bothersome, isolating them like caged animals, and then medicating them with soporific drugs from the midtwentieth century and without the benefit of advancements from the past seven decades of revolutionary medical research. The truth is I've not *learned* this. We all *know* this. Instead, through documenting this crisis, I've been forced to come to terms with what is right in front of us all—visible on the streets and in our own families.

To make sense of the current state of our mental health care system, I've spoken with hundreds of people about SMI and SED, including their family members, and the world's experts. But I knew that to truly understand and explain, I had to begin at home.

CHAPTER I

HOW IT ALL BEGAN

It had been two weeks since I'd spoken to Merle, and I was afraid. For months, I'd been calling my sister every few days, cajoling, threatening, using every carrot and stick I could to convince her to move to a facility that could care for her and where she might make friends for the first time in decades. Finally, she'd stopped answering the phone. Now fifty-five years old, she had been living on her own for the first time since my mother had died two years earlier.

On December 27, 2005, after fourteen days of silence, I rode the Metro North train home from work in my Manhattan office, focused on the task ahead. As an addiction psychiatrist, I had spent the day treating people with depression, anxiety, and drug and alcohol problems. Over the years, I had received many notes of thanks from patients for saving their lives from their various addictions. But it had been years since I treated someone for schizophrenia.

I lived a comfortable life, commuting between my Upper East Side office and a bedroom community in Scarsdale. The loving and stable home I'd created with my wife and our two children offered a complete departure from my chaotic childhood in Philadelphia. Now the chaos was creeping back in. Despite all my psychiatric training and practice, I was at a loss for what to do about my sister. As the only other surviving member of our family, I was the last person left to care for her. Cancer had taken my father first, and later my eldest sister, Gail. Finally, my mother's passing left me in charge.

I had been determined to find a reasonable plan for Merle's well-being and had made arrangements with a convalescent home that could offer her a life free from the years of hoarding that had turned the house where we grew up into a hovel. But the longer my calls went unanswered, the clearer it became that I would have to betray my mother's dying wish that I never, ever call the police on my sister.

I walked the mile from the train station to my home and dialed Merle yet again, picturing the beige telephone that sat on the island separating the kitchen from the living room, where as a child, I'd often watched TV while we ate dinner. I pictured the black phone that sat on the night table next to my parents' bed—the big bed, the comfortable bed, the bed on which I'd jumped and played, the only bed near a TV, in the room with a bright view of the street—the room where Merle had recovered after her accident, the room where we'd had one of our worst fights, the room where she now slept.

I knew that even if I could get the police to take Merle to a hospital, it would be nearly impossible to keep her there for long. I was well acquainted with the commitment laws, which dictate that you can't involuntarily hospitalize someone unless they declare themselves to be immediately suicidal or homicidal to an impartial evaluating psychiatrist. One of the few exceptions in some states is when a doctor swears that a patient is so incapacitated that they can't feed themselves—not even at a shelter or by scavenging through garbage cans the way the estimated 194,000 unsheltered homeless and the 552,000 total homeless people do every day in

America.[1] Otherwise, it's illegal to admit someone to a locked facility for more than a few days of observation. I had heard there were ways to petition the court so that a relative could assume control, but that would require supporting paperwork, a court hearing, and a judge's determination. Pursuing that course was certain to incur Merle's wrath, but I was running out of options.

It was not unusual for Merle to avoid me. In the two years since my mother's death, I had often called the emergency operator, who would report that the phone was off the hook. "Call the police?" they would suggest. *No police*, I thought. My sister would call me when she was ready. But this time was different; the phone was on the receiver.

In a last-ditch effort to avoid the unavoidable, I reached out to Gail's widower, my brother-in-law Bob, who lived nearby, to ask him to knock on the door. No answer. Mail was piled on the doorstep. It was time to make the call.

• • •

As Gail told it, Merle was an irascible child. Gail was six years old when Merle was born and recalled my parents struggling to manage the baby, trying in vain to get her to lie down in her crib. I was born six years later, and for as long as I can remember, Merle was prone to erupting at any moment, lashing out at my mother or at Gail, if she happened to be home (once she moved out to attend Temple University in downtown Philly, that wasn't often). I had always been in awe of Gail—my cool, blond sister who had breezed in and out of our house between boyfriends and adventures—but we didn't really connect until years later, as Merle's condition declined and we joined forces against our parents' denial.

Over the years, arguments between Merle and my mother grew louder and became physical. As a small child, I would scream at the top of my lungs, briefly producing a cease-fire. That strategy worked, until it didn't. Then only my dad could make them stop. When Merle's rage escalated, my mother would telephone my father over and over, summoning him home from work, pleading for help. Sometimes she would pull me to the phone to corroborate that Merle was "impossible" and he had to come. My father was a tough guy from South Philly, never one to back down from a fight. Merle taunted him to no end.

When Merle's teenage fury morphed into adult psychosis, her illness became our family's Watergate, a scandal to cover up at any cost. To my working-class Jewish parents, any mental illness was a *shanda*, Yiddish for "disgrace." They had come of age before the discovery of the new antipsychotic drugs in 1950, and their expectations were likely colored by what they had heard about the so-called snake-pit hospitals of their generation, a reputation dating back to the very first lunatic asylum, Bedlam.

• • •

A word now synonymous with disorder and mayhem, Bedlam was the colloquial name of England's Bethlem Hospital, which was founded as a priory in 1247 and has cared for "lunatics" from 1377 to the present day.[2] In *A Foreign View of England* (1902), César de Saussure described conditions at the hospital like this:

> You find yourself in a long and wide gallery, on either
> side of which are a large number of little cells where
> lunatics of every description are shut up, and you can
> get a sight of these poor creatures, little windows being

let into the doors. Many inoffensive madmen walk in the big gallery. On the second floor is a corridor and cells like those on the first floor, and this is the part reserved for dangerous maniacs, most of them being chained and terrible to behold.[3]

Bethlem, the nearby village, had been a quiet backwater until the 1630s, when it became a bustling center. Close as it was to "the first Elizabethan theaters and other sources of entertainment," Bedlam, the hospital, evolved into a sightseeing destination where the public was welcome to ogle the patients—for a fee. In the seventeenth and eighteenth centuries, explain the authors of *The History of Bethlem*, "casual visitors contributed quite substantial sums to the income of the Hospital and its staff."[4]

According to Roy Porter, a historian whom I've admired since med school and author of *Mind-Forg'd Manacles: A History of Madness in England from the Restoration to the Regency*, this open-door policy may have fed the hospital's ill repute:

> Spectators thronged to see unaccommodated man. And largely because Bethlem housed the only collection of mad-people in the nation, it achieved a sort of concentrated notoriety; it became an epitome of all that people fantasized about madness itself. All this conspired to give Bethlem its lasting dubious reputation. At best conveying gloomy horoscope, it symbolized the revenue of natural man—Chaos come again.[5]

What "most discredits Bethlem," according to Porter, was "its lasting practical therapeutic apathy" whereby those charged with patient care advanced neither research about insanity nor its treatment.[6] Indeed, not until the seventeenth century did the hospital even retain medical professionals,[7] and once it did, the "curative" approaches reflected the misinformation and barbarism of the age.

Here in the United States, the treatment approaches were not much better. In colonial times, madness was considered symptomatic of a spiritual or moral failing and was thought to stem from both natural and supernatural causes, including demonic possession. These illnesses were cause for scorn, punishment, or both. If they didn't end up in almshouses or jails, most people with mental diseases were cared for by family members. The few treatments available included bloodletting and purging (aka evacuating the bowels of) those afflicted.

The first "organized effort to care for the mentally ill" in America, according to the U.S. National Library of Medicine, was made by Philadelphia Quakers in 1752 when they set up a cluster of basement rooms equipped with shackles that could accommodate a small number of patients in Pennsylvania Hospital.[8] Within two years, in response to increased demand, they expanded to a freestanding ward next door. The facility, which moved to a new location and changed its name, was among America's first mental institutions, setting the stage for a new phase in treatment: institutional care.

Although the nineteenth century brought about few advancements in the scientific understanding of psychiatric disorders, profound changes in public perception shaped different priorities for care.[9] Spearheading this transformation was Dorothea Dix, who, from 1843 on, campaigned on behalf of the "helpless, forgotten, insane, and idiotic men and women; of beings, sunk to a condition from which the most unconcerned would start with real horror."[10] Perhaps the best-known early advocate for "moral treatment," Dix argued that instead of locking people away in almshouses or jails, small, "*rightly organized Hospitals*, adapted to the special care of the peculiar malady of the Insane," could "re-educate" ill individuals. Offering occupational therapy, religious exercises, amusements, and games could promote healing.[11] Dix petitioned state legislatures, on moral grounds, to commit funds toward institutions that would offer attentive, individualized care. This led virtually every state to establish one or more public hospitals, launching a century-long practice of state responsibility for the care and treatment of people with mental illness.[12]

In keeping with the values of the times, some private mental hospitals adopted programs of exercise and recreation that included concerts and dances called "lunatic balls."[13] (In the late nineteenth century, a state hospital in Middletown, New York, even established a men's baseball team, with each player wearing a uniform emblazoned with the name "Asylum."[14]) In 1856, Pennsylvania Hospital founded the independent Pennsylvania Hospital for the Insane, which promoted "moral treatment" rooted in the belief that mental illness could be cured by respectful care in a wholesome environment.[15]

In contrast to the earlier warehouses that locked patients in filthy, crowded wards, often in chains, it set a new standard of care with spacious, airy quarters where residents had private rooms and spent time outdoors, attended lectures, and visited the hospital library. Pennsylvania Hospital was also where my sister received care after she suffered her first psychotic break at age twenty, and it provided me with my first glimpse of psychiatric treatment.

• • •

Merle had a quick and creative mind and laughed at the silliest of jokes. With her wide smile, my sister was, it seemed to me, as personable and funny as our favorite television star, Carol Burnett. Sometimes she would entertain me by performing one-woman comedy skits fashioned after Burnett's show in the doorway of my bedroom. Merle always belted out a song as her grand finale. My favorite was her rendition of "Sunny" and, like a fan at a concert, I'd call out for it and she'd oblige. "More, more!" I'd cry out as Merle took a bow. If I was lucky, she might tell a one-liner or sing another tune. I was Merle's adoring audience.

To me, Merle was also as pretty as could be. But she always worried that boys weren't interested in her. At age nineteen, she met her first boyfriend, another freshman at a small college nearby in New Jersey. A year later, they were married. The wedding was a rushed affair, held on the heels of Gail's wedding—the following year, at the same synagogue, with the same caterer.

Marriage seemed to offer progress toward the future she dreamed of: becoming a wife, a mother, and a schoolteacher. But within a year, their newlywed arguments grew hostile and Merle and her husband split up. Their marriage was annulled, and with that my sister's first, and only, romantic relationship was erased as if it had never happened.

Merle returned home bereft, hysterical. It's impossible to say whether the breakup was precipitated by early symptoms of mental illness or if her grief triggered a rapid decline. There's a dynamic flux between factors—that is, mental illness doesn't just happen in a vacuum. There's a progression of illness, exacerbated by life's stresses, during which the smoldering brain erupts into an all-out, five-alarm fire.

My sister's challenges with relationships and her generalized anxieties were signs that a bigger problem might be looming. Psychological treatment and judicious use of medications for at-risk behaviors might have prevented worse problems down the road. But that's not what happened. Hoping to make a fresh start, Merle went off to a different college. By the end of the fall semester in her second year, she was failing out of school. She was entering what I now know to be the prodromal phase of psychosis, which included magical thinking, poor judgment, bad anxiety, mood shifts, self-imposed isolation, and strange behavior that was inconsistent with her earlier life. Psychiatrists will tell you that minimizing stress and avoiding substances of abuse, which is particularly challenging for many college students, is essential during this prodrome period. But it was hard for Merle—and us—to reduce stress while everyone was busy minimizing the disaster that was brewing. The following year, it became unavoidable.

I was fourteen when my sister transformed into someone unrecognizable. Once, a new college friend telephoned to say that he was worried that she was out of touch with reality. My parents dismissed him as a jilted lover, but Gail knew better—even before Merle's condition deteriorated to the worst we'd ever seen.

Months later, Merle was visiting Gail at her downtown apartment. The two stayed up talking long after Gail's husband, Bob, who had to get up early for work, went to bed. At around two in the morning, Gail shook him awake in a panic. "Get up," Gail urged. "You gotta come out here and listen to this." Merle was hallucinating and paranoid. She didn't recognize them. Bob and Gail did their best to calm her down and everyone went to sleep. But by morning, Merle had disappeared.

Gail and Bob finally found her down the block in a phone booth, railing, frightened, and still unable to recognize them. Bob was reluctant to touch her or to try to pull her out. Wanting to take her someplace that could help, somewhere "appropriate," as Bob later told me, he called his internist, who gave him the name of a psychiatrist, who suggested Pennsylvania Hospital.

Meanwhile Merle was still holed up, babbling the high-speed speech of psychosis, clearly terrified by her new sense of reality. When they couldn't convince her to come out, Bob and Gail called the police. Two officers arrived with a van and put her in the back. In a moment of kindness, they let Bob and Gail ride with Merle since she was so frightened, and also agreed to bend the rule mandating that they go to the nearest hospital in order to bring her to Forty-eighth and Market Street, where the psychiatrist Bob had spoken with was waiting. Bob had only ever heard "Forty-eighth and Market Street" used as a pejorative: the building that held Philly's lunatics. Now he was delivering his sister-in-law to its gates.

This was Merle's earliest full break with reality. That she had been brought, safely, to a reputable facility meant that she was far luckier than most people confronting their first episode of psychosis. It was early enough in her disease that the psychological trauma, social alienation, and possible biological deterioration of the brain caused by extended psychosis could probably have been prevented. *Maybe if she had stayed hospitalized, the doctors could have devised a long-term treatment plan. Maybe she'd have come to understand that she was sick and needed medicine. Maybe her downward spiral could have even been reversed.*

Merle stayed for a week or so, during which my family participated in a handful of family therapy sessions, seated in a semicircle of sofas and chairs. I thought the psychiatrist seemed like a cool guy, with a bicycle and an office full of books. I felt at home in his office. He had a way of understanding the newly blossoming hallucinations. He spoke about the unspeakable—about the denial, anger, avoidance, and blaming that I witnessed in my household.

He granted me and Gail the chance to participate in an open dialogue about our family life—a platform to plead our case. The psychiatrist answered my prayers for understanding, interpreting our family's story as the consequence of a serious medical disease. Merle wasn't "impossible." She was sick and needed help. My parents weren't bad parents. In fact, they were as dedicated as they came. My folks were just terrified.

I learned through Merle's hospitalization that there was a name for her illness: schizophrenia (although, given the range of her symptoms in mood, thought, personality, and anxiety, the actual, complete diagnosis remains unclear to me to this day). That her craziness had a name reassured me. Maybe that meant there was a way to fix it.

Schizophrenia is a psychotic disorder that affects someone's sense of what's real, causing changes in how they think, act, and feel. The disease is characterized by both "positive" and "negative" symptoms. The positive symptoms—hallucinations (hearing or seeing things) and delusions (unreal and magical thoughts)—are most evident in the beginning stages of the illness, while the negative symptoms of apathy, isolation, withdrawal, and poor thinking ability come to the fore later. These "positive" symptoms of dysfunctional thinking make schizophrenia a "thought disorder" as opposed to a "mood disorder" like depression or bipolar disorder. The speech patterns of schizophrenia often include rhyming and nonsense words. This disjointed, erratic, nonsensical language use is referred to as *word salad*. Psychiatrists once thought a schizophrenia diagnosis—generally a disease that develops during young adulthood—meant a serious downward course toward a future that would preclude work, romantic relationships, or functioning independently. Nowadays, however, we have increasingly come to recognize that many people with the disease lead full, productive lives, particularly if it is treated early and continuously. That was not to be the case for Merle.

During our few family therapy sessions, Merle was livid. She paced back and forth, yelling that hospital staff were forcing her to take drugs that were hurting her, that they were manhandling her and forcing her into the shower. Still, wanting desperately to believe that the madness would resolve when Merle left the madhouse, my parents insisted nothing was wrong with her.

When Gail and I told Merle that she belonged in the hospital, she snapped at us, "*You* belong here! *You're* the crazy ones!" She blamed us for creating a charade of mental illness that would subject her to harmful treatments. Nothing Gail or I said made a difference—especially not once the psychiatrist started asking personal questions that pushed my parents over the edge.

In the 1970s, many psychiatrists believed mental illness could be understood through psychoanalytic or Freudian techniques. Freud believed that neurotic illnesses were a function of sexual traumas during critical stages of development (not sexual abuse but subtle disturbances in normal development, like the famous Oedipal complex, in which prepubescent boys feel an intense connection to their mothers and a threat from their fathers). Psychoanalysts believed that through offering insightful interpretations, they could get the patient to understand, accept, and change themselves. Many extended the Freudian concepts to understand and treat people with psychosis and SMI. The approach was not without merit, but timing is everything. Immediately following Merle's first hospitalization, my whole family was shell-shocked. This was not the time to dig too deeply into my wounded family's unconscious.

As my sister paced back and forth, ranting, the doctor asked my parents if they made love in their bedroom, and if we, their children, ever heard them. It was undeniably an odd question, but then again, the whole experience felt surreal. Mom obediently answered that she was afraid to have sex when the children were around, but Dad wouldn't dignify the question with an answer. I don't think the psychiatrist meant any harm. It was just one of dozens of questions he asked to try to understand the family dynamics in an era when psychiatrists believed that sexual problems were important in understanding the genesis of mental illness. Now I understand my dad's outrage at the intrusive question, especially asked while his kids—all of us angry with him—looked on, and while his wife sobbed, pleading with him to let her take Merle home.

Gail's and my defending the doctor made things worse. A take-charge man, Dad lashed out. No longer would he permit his children's insubordination. In his view, the lunatics were running the asylum and look where it had gotten us. His daughter was being held captive and was claiming that male attendants were manhandling her in the shower. His wife was crying nonstop and seeking answers where none existed. "You are no longer in charge," Dad scolded us.

"We were never in charge," I yelled back.

It was the first time I'd dared take on my dad. Seizing upon the psychiatrist's permission to think psychologically, I said that the very fact that we couldn't have a calm discussion in this office was evidence enough that Gail and I didn't run a thing. If we'd been in charge, I argued, we would have begun family therapy years earlier and Merle would have been hospitalized long ago.

That session was our last. Against medical advice and Gail's and my protests, Merle came home. It was at that moment that I decided to become a psychiatrist.

At fourteen, I hadn't the slightest interest in science. Nor did I fully appreciate that becoming a psychiatrist would entail a decade-long training commitment including attending medical school, completing an internship, and spending three more years of training in my psychiatry specialty, and then two more years in fellowship for subspecialization. All I knew was that to my parents, the psychiatrist was the enemy, and I was ready and willing to enlist in his army. As a teenager, I started reading books about psychotherapy and mental illness, beginning with Freud. I also read Freud's critics, like Thomas Szasz, as well as humanist psychiatrists who compellingly challenged conventional psychiatric practices. I attended psychology seminars, went to readings and movies about mental illness, and began individual therapy to try to understand myself and my world better. All the while, I kept the family secret—even from my therapist. When he asked about my interest in psychiatry, I told him that I wanted to know more about the intersection of brain and mind. I never told a single person about my sister—not even my best friends.

After Merle left the hospital, my parents sought the counsel of a respected Philadelphia psychiatrist. (The pull of denial was strong, but my parents were no fools.) By my mother's account, he had little to offer but pity, telling her that such cases broke his heart. When my sister's behavior got particularly out of hand, my parents arranged for another hospitalization. At sixteen years old, I got my driver's license and became the designated driver to take Merle to the hospital. But these episodes of treatment were always short-lived and interspersed with periods where my parents convinced themselves that nothing was wrong with Merle. At one point, my mother reached out to my grandmother's former internist, who was now a psychiatrist working at the nearby Friends Hospital. I drove

Merle to her third hospitalization where, under this trusted doctor's care, my parents permitted her to receive ten electroshock treatments over the course of several weeks. Merle left the hospital determined to never go back.

Beyond that determination, her inpatient stay offered one other lasting outcome: the doctor began giving Merle monthly injections of an antipsychotic medication called Prolixin that would last a full month. The drug caused terrible drowsiness for days, messed up Merle's endocrine system, and made her gain more than fifty pounds. But it also reduced the intensity of the voices and delusions and made her life more manageable. Even she couldn't deny that it was helping, and she stuck with those injections for the rest of her life.

Still, Merle never held a job, went back to school, or made a new friend. She wanted nothing to do with clubhouses where people with schizophrenia and similar disorders congregate and support one other. She avoided individual and group therapy, and any place where there were "crazy people." My dad immersed himself in work and spent more time away from home. Given that no cures were forthcoming, Merle, like many people with psychiatric disorders, refused any treatment aside from the Prolixin injections. Instead, she stayed in her room, praying for it all to stop.

A few months after I started college as a premed student, I came home late one night to find everyone gone. The phone rang and the voice on the other end told me I needed to come to the hospital immediately. Merle had fallen from her bedroom window onto the concrete driveway three stories below. The neighbors had found her screaming. I found her shattered, twisted glasses on the table downstairs. At the ICU, I learned that she had broken many of the major bones in her body.

How she had managed to do this remains beyond my comprehension. Had voices commanded her to end it all? Did those voices transmit a message of self-loathing—the culmination of four years of family denial that she was sick, of the pain of her annulment, of winding up a college dropout despite all her hard work? Or had she heard something that had spooked her? The sound of our heavy doorknocker, perhaps—a salesman or someone asking for directions? Ultimately, maybe she was just beset with what people with her problem constantly face: a world of unimaginable sensory experiences coupled with a complete lack of judgment.

I have since learned that jumping from windows is common among people experiencing a psychotic break. Rather than being a suicide attempt per se, it often stems from an urgent need to escape. In approximately 80 percent of cases, the jump seems to have been impulsive.[16] It accounts for roughly 25 percent of suicides and occurs most commonly among single women early in the course of their psychotic disease.[17] But all I knew at the time was that at age twenty-four, Merle's fall would chart the course of her life, which would now be forever constrained—a life so unlike Gail's: at the time, she had a four-year-old, a kind husband, and a town house in downtown Philadelphia. A life so unlike mine: her little brother was on track to become a doctor and have a family. A life unlike our parents': at the moment she jumped, they had been celebrating at the wedding of the child of a family friend.

In the aftermath, my parents sought out the leading surgeons at the University of Pennsylvania. When it came to bodily ailments, my parents were devoted caretakers who followed the doctors' orders precisely. Although they had modest means, they spared no expense to help Merle recover. My father kept a vigil for weeks at her bedside, sleeping in the hospital room so someone would be there day and night. The surgeons and nurses who treated her held hero status in our family. My father, who worked in the wholesale meat business, brought them steaks.

When Merle came home, my parents turned their bedroom into a rehabilitation center. My mother devoted all her attention to Merle's physical needs, and no task was too burdensome, including changing bedpans. Miraculously, Merle emerged (physically) whole, save for some well-hidden facial scars, a slight limp, flexion problems in her wrist, and immobility in her fingers that led her to use the back of her hand to push up her glasses when they slid down her nose. Whatever had led her to jump was never discussed.

In the months that followed, an employee of my father's—a carpenter and electrician who was at the house making some repairs—said to me out of the blue, "You know, they really should catch people like that and cut off their—"

"What are you talking about?" I asked, fully confused.

I don't remember his exact words, but he said something to the effect of "You know, the guy who came into your house and tried to get your sister." That's how I learned about the cover story my father had concocted—a tale that transformed my parents' denial and shame over my sister's mental illness into a tale of her bravery and virtue. I said nothing.

Through contacts I'd made in the psychology department at the local college, I found a psychologist and a psychiatrist both willing to visit Merle at home. But there was to be no sustained treatment beyond the shots. Looking back, I understand my parents' reluctance and skepticism. Although the surgeons had tools that were able to return Merle to some semblance of normalcy, psychiatric care could not restore her mind. There was also the societal stigma to contend with, and the fact that my parents never approached psychiatric care with the same respect and spirit of collaboration that they granted to the surgeons. And so, despite the resources they mustered to support her physical care, the shame combined with the paucity of effective solutions prevented Merle from receiving truly therapeutic treatment. Instead, her illness kept running the show and ultimately all of our lives.

Two years after her fall, Merle could walk. Finally, I could run. I was no longer needed to help out my bedridden sister and my sorrowful mother. Gail, my beacon of sanity, urged me on, and I wore down my parents until they agreed to let me leave home. After two years at the local college, I was leaving home to spend my last two years of college in Boston.

In the early-morning hours one day in August 1976, while my family slept, I loaded up the AMC Eagle hatchback my father had bought me. When I turned the key in the ignition, the Little Feat song "All That You Dream" came on WMMR. Merle often said that the car radio telepathically communicated to her, but now the radio station seemed to be helping *me!* My new favorite band, Little Feat, inspiring me to hightail it out of there and pursue my own dreams! I backed down the driveway and pointed my car north, tears streaming down my face. *Finally . . . I was free.*

• • •

Years later I would meet many others like me—people who had come to the practice of psychiatry through their experiences with family members struggling with mental health issues. Among them was Fuller Torrey, MD, a research psychiatrist whom I met at a watershed moment in my life. By 2005, Merle, Gail, and my parents had all died. With the incredible help of my wife, I soldiered on with the formalities of a dutiful brother: giving the eulogies and buying the headstones. I steered clear of Philadelphia, focusing on my kids and building up my academic life and medical practice. Yet those traumatic years around Merle's death and the loss of my family of origin took an enormous toll on our twenty-five-year marriage. Six years after Merle's death, in 2011, my wife and I began divorce proceedings. Although we've remained the best of friends, the split shook me to the core. The secure nest that I had created—the antidote to the chaos of my upbringing—had vanished. Memories of Merle came flooding back with a vengeance.

With the dissolution of my close-knit family unit, I was set adrift at the same age when both my sisters had died. I decided I had to do something to make a difference for families like mine before time ran out. I wanted to document the mental health crisis in this country and wondered how I should go about it. I emailed the world's foremost expert: Dr. Torrey.

One night, while I was driving home from the gym, the phone rang. I pulled over on a dark road not far from Long Island Sound. During that call, and over the years through our many long conversations, Dr. Torrey became my guide, helping me see that SMI was not just my own family's struggle but the greatest social crisis of our time.

Dr. Torrey had been a junior at Princeton when his mother found his eighteen-year-old sister Rhoda hallucinating in the front yard.[18] Those early signs of confusion escalated into delusions and hearing voices, and soon Rhoda was diagnosed with schizophrenia.[19] He accompanied his mother as she brought Rhoda to all the best institutions for the available treatments, including the dangerous insulin coma therapies, in which a hypoglycemic coma was induced by injections of insulin. She spent much of the rest of her life in hospitals, community group homes, and finally a nursing home, where she died at age seventy of pulmonary disease.

Decades prior, doctors had told Dr. Torrey's mother that Rhoda had developed the disease in part because Dr. Torrey's father had died when their children were young.[20] Their mother spent her entire life believing that she had somehow caused his sister's illness. At the time a common theory prevailed that "schizophrenogenic mothers"—said to be overprotective, or rejecting, or just "toxic"— caused the disease.[21] Even if doctors didn't point a finger directly, many mothers did that on their own. Many still do. Whenever a child is suffering, most parents naturally have questions: *Did I miss the signs? What could I have done better?* And the dreaded *Did I do anything to cause this?* The blame game has always been alive and well in mental health. *Whose fault is this?* we ask, looking for a villain, even among the victims. (Today, we often blame the professionals who are called in to help—nurses, doctors, first responders such as EMTs—and anyone else who fails in healing the sick.)

Surely bad parenting can harm children, but no research shows that even the worst parenting causes psychosis. "I developed a sneaking suspicion that these eminent psychiatrists did not know what they were talking about," Dr. Torrey later explained.[22] He came to believe that SMI might instead be caused by genetics or viruses, or likely a combination of biological inclination and environmental forces.

After earning his medical degree, Dr. Torrey trained in psychiatry at Stanford University and went on to become the nation's foremost medical professional who advocates for people with SMI. In 1998, he founded the Treatment Advocacy Center (TAC), a group aimed at eliminating legal and other barriers to treatment.[23] He has written twenty books, leading to public criticism of his calls for forced treatment for those who are too sick to recognize their illness, and he incurred professional criticism for unabashedly calling out psychiatry for not doing enough to help people like Rhoda.

Dr. Torrey is a renegade who asks the most incisive and critical questions of our time, essential to understanding America's mental health crisis: *Why does our country allow these people to languish in jail and on the streets? Why have the past few decades seen so few significant medical or research advancements or any real advocacy toward improvements in care? Why do we allow sick people who don't know they're sick to reject treatment?* He sees our abandonment of people with SMI as a "150-year-old disaster." That night on the telephone, Dr. Torrey agreed to advise me on my quest to understand the lives of Americans with SMI. He told me that grasping the genesis of the problem meant unpacking the history of deinstitutionalization and the social history of our country.

• • •

Many people blame President Reagan. A few blame President Kennedy. Some people blame the doctors and pharmaceutical companies. Some people blame conservatives and those on the right for wanting to lock people away in horrible asylums. Some blame the left-leaning civil libertarians for blocking institutionalization and championing the freethinking outpatient centers that were never capable of caring for the truly sick patents. As far as I'm concerned, there are no villains, just many victims. Most of the providers of mental health care have meant well, and it doesn't solve our mental health crisis to lapse into the popular pastime of the who's-to-blame game when the essential problem does not lie with any institution, body politic, or group of doctors. The real problem is the illness: the poorly understood and insufficiently treated illness. With that caveat, I want to take you on a brief tour of how and why we have managed to make a very bad situation worse over the past one-hundred-plus years.

Since med school, I've been fascinated by the history of psychiatric medicine, particularly the period that historians call the era of "great and desperate cures."[24] Some notable treatments over the years have included the following:

- Focal infection therapy (1910s): removing teeth, the pancreas, ovaries, and/or parts of the colon based on the notion that silent infections in these tissues caused insanity

- Insulin coma therapy (early 1930s to 1940s): weeks and months spent chemically inducing a temporary coma on a daily basis, which sometimes brought about seizures from hefty insulin injections, based on the idea that the brain needed to rest and reset

- Electroconvulsive therapy (ECT) (late 1930s to present): applying an electrical current to the forehead to bring about seizures in an attempt to reset the brain (by the 1960s, ECT would become extremely effective for certain conditions when done properly, *with* anesthesia)

- Leucotomy (aka frontal lobotomy) (late 1930s to 1950s): hammering an ice-pick-like instrument through the eye socket to reach the brain and then blindly chiseling away brain tissue from the supposed emotional connections in the frontal lobes

The most instructive story is that of lobotomy, which would ultimately be performed on tens of thousands of people after it was developed by Egas Moniz, MD. In a clear demonstration of just how desperate we were to find anything resembling a cure for SMI, the barbaric procedure earned Dr. Moniz Portugal's and psychiatry's first

Nobel Prize in medicine in 1949. Some doctors urged that this irre-versible surgery be performed as early as possible in the course of the illness before the brain deteriorated further. Among those loboto-mized was President John F. Kennedy's sister, Rosemary. In his book *American Psychosis*, Dr. Torrey connects the historical dots between Rosemary Kennedy's condition and subsequent lobotomy, JFK's sense of moral responsibility, and the transformation of federal policy regarding the asylum and treatment of SMI.[25] Through Rosemary, Dr. Torrey says that President Kennedy learned firsthand the horrors of the state-of-the-art care.

Rose Kennedy realized early on that her "very pretty baby" Rose-mary was not developing as expected. Rosemary's developmental delays kept her from advancing to first grade, and even with inten-sive tutoring she was unable to ever progress beyond a fourth-grade level in math or a fifth-grade level in English.[26] By the summer of 1939, when Rosemary was twenty-one, symptoms of mental illness appeared. Two years later, as Doris Kearns Goodwin explains in *The Fitzgeralds and the Kennedys*, Rosemary began lashing out with "tantrums, rages, and violent behavior . . . like a wild animal, given to screaming, cursing, and thrashing out at anyone who tried to thwart her will."[27]

By the time Rosemary was a young adult with a combination of mental retardation and severe behavioral disturbances, her behavior grew increasingly troublesome, and her parents grew more desperate for a solution. The neurologist Walter J. Freeman, MD, who became notorious for traveling from hospital to hospital in a station wagon with his ice-pick-like instruments for lobotomy, performed the pro-cedure with neurosurgeon James W. Watts, MD. In his book *The Sins of the Father*, Ronald Kessler shares Dr. Watts's account of the pro-cedure: After mildly sedating Rosemary and drilling two small holes in the top of her skull, Watts inserted a knife and "swung it up and down to cut brain tissue . . . As Dr. Watts cut, Dr. Freeman asked Rosemary questions. For example, he asked her to recite the Lord's Prayer or to sing 'God Bless America' or count backward . . . 'We made an estimate on how far to cut based on how she responded,' Dr. Watts said. When she began to become incoherent, they stopped."[28]

The once lively woman emerged from the surgery no longer able to wash or dress herself. And she had also lost most of her ability to speak. Although she seemed to understand others, she was unable to respond and spent hours staring at the wall.[29] She lived out her days institutionalized. Rosemary's horrific ordeal, Dr. Torrey told me, laid the groundwork for today's epidemic, as the son tried to atone for the sins of the father.

JFK would become the president who cemented deinstitutionalization. But even before Kennedy's presidency, America's asylums had already become a national embarrassment. In 1946, *Life* magazine published the game-changing exposé "BEDLAM 1946: Most of the U.S. Mental Hospitals Are a Shame and Disgrace." The investigative piece centered on the Philadelphia State Hospital at Byberry, a short bike ride from my childhood home. Constructed during the early twentieth century's wave of state-of-the-art facilities offering rest and cure, it had, along with other asylums in the country, devolved by midcentury. This article echoed and animated a shift in public opinion away from institutionalization in favor of outpatient care.

Change was afoot in government as well. In 1945, the chief of the Mental Hygiene Division of the Mental Health Service, Robert H. Felix, MD, was charged by the surgeon general with developing a comprehensive national mental health program. That effort led to the establishment of NIMH one year later. When Dr. Felix took the helm as the agency's first director, he said his aim was "to employ the prestige and resources of the national government to redirect mental health priorities"—a radical and virtually unprecedented declaration for the time.[30] With the bill establishing NIMH signed into law in 1946, the federal government officially committed to providing mental health care to its citizens. Two years later, Dr. Felix awarded $2.1 million to forty-five states "for assistance in the development or expansion of community mental health services."[31] With this, the movement to nationalize mental health care was launched.

A decade later, lobbying efforts spearheaded by Dr. Felix were operating in full force. To generate public support and lay the groundwork for the establishment of a comprehensive national program, Dr. Felix pushed for a Joint Commission on Mental Illness and Health to hold congressional hearings and create a report. Predictably, that report made recommendations drawn from Dr. Felix's long-standing opinions that state mental hospitals were utterly bankrupt of therapeutic value and should be abolished, and that psychiatric illnesses could be treated in the community with no need for inpatient care. "Public mental hospitals as we know them today can disappear," he said, because "all the various types of emotionally disturbed patients can be handled in the community."[32] Although the commission's report was completed by early 1959, Dr. Felix and his colleagues stalled its publication until they knew the results of the 1960 presidential election. As soon as JFK was elected, they released it, confident that they now had a sympathetic audience in the White House. Kennedy was indeed sympathetic, and his concerns were buoyed by a groundswell of disillusionment about state institutions as well as a growing belief among psychiatrists that outpatient care could offer effective treatment.

The emergence of the antipsychotic medicine chlorpromazine seemed to present further evidence. Chlorpromazine, which had been developed in France in 1952, originally for potential use in anesthesia, was marketed in the United States under the trade name Thorazine. It significantly reduced delusions, hallucinations, and mania in patients with psychosis. Pharmacological relief was a significant breakthrough, enabling many people to leave the hospitals to which they had been consigned, possibly for a lifetime.[33] Given the breakthroughs of the day, President Kennedy likely expected that scientists would discover even better medicines to eliminate the scourge of mental illness and make the run-down asylums obsolete once and for all.

These factors converged with the passage of the Community Mental Health Acts of 1963 and 1965, which, as Gerald N. Grob and Howard H. Goldman, MD, PhD, explain in *The Dilemma of Federal Mental Health Policy*, "had two basic objectives: first, to replace archaic and obsolete mental hospitals that had presumably outlived their usefulness; second, to create a radically new institution—the community mental health center—that would benefit individuals with severe and persistent mental disorders."[34]

On February 5, 1963, President Kennedy presented the bill in a historic "Special Message" to Congress in which he described state hospitals and homes as "shamefully understaffed, overcrowded, unpleasant institutions from which death too often provided the only firm hope of release."[35] As a humane alternative, he called for outpatient clinics. Now, more than fifty years later, JFK's words of optimism and hope still speak to me:

Almost every family at some stage will experience, or has experienced, a case of mental affliction. And we have to offer something more than crowded custodial care in our state institutions. Our task is to prevent these conditions. Our next is to treat them more effectively and sympathetically in the patient's own community.[36]

Kennedy envisioned a future where people with mental illness would no longer live in shame and isolation. Carrying out the act's recommendations would transform mental health care so that "reliance on the cold mercy of custodial isolation will be supplanted by the open warmth of community concern and capability."[37]

As Grob and Goldman point out, "The decline of traditional mental hospital care and the rise of a community care policy, paradoxically, created a fragmented rather than a unified mental health system. Those most in need—persons with severe disorders—have often proved to be the losers."[38] The passage of the Community Mental Health Act signified a substantial shift in American mental health policy.[39] Yet the amendments to the Social Security Act championed by Lyndon Johnson, who became president in 1963, wound up having even more profound effects on mental health care delivery through the creation of Medicare and Medicaid. As Richard G. Frank and Sherry A. Glied explain in *Better but Not Well*, Medicaid, which helps cover medical costs for some people with limited income and resources, "allowed beneficiaries to purchase mental health care from any provider willing to accept Medicaid fees as payment in full. . . . Enrollees with mental disorders were, for the first time, able to choose among general hospital psychiatric units, community health centers, outpatient mental health clinics, and, to a more limited extent, office-based psychiatrists and psychologists."[40]

Aside from providing this array of care choices to a previously underserved population, these amendments cemented the transition away from both state and private mental hospitals by specifically excluding these large institutions from Medicaid payment. The Institution of Mental Disease (IMD) exclusion specified that any hospital or health facility that allotted more than sixteen beds to mental health care would be denied Medicaid payment. This exclusion would become one of the most hotly contested issues in mental health care, a debate that continues to this day.

In 1955, there were 558,922 psychiatric patients in state mental hospitals.[41] A year later, that number had dropped by 7,532, in what Dr. Torrey called "the first such decrease in more than a century."[42] In a nation where state hospitals were once the primary source of care for people with SMI—many of whom spent their lives in these facilities—deinstitutionalization was well under way. Yet of the two thousand community mental health centers proposed to replace the demolished asylums, only half wound up being built and those were only partly funded. This last piece of legislation signed by President Kennedy before his assassination created a sweeping plan for mental health care that he never had the opportunity to see through. By the 1980s, fewer than one hundred of the outpatient community mental health centers that were built to solve America's mental illness crisis remained.

Dr. Torrey told me that the United States currently has just 2 to 3 percent of the psychiatric treatment beds that we had sixty years ago: "We now have so few beds available for people with mental illness that there's nowhere to put them." Because emergency departments are legally required to treat anyone who comes through the door, people with SMI often wind up staying there for days or even weeks at a time waiting for a psychiatric treatment bed. We see that across the country. But which single hospital would best show us the crisis?

• • •

"Go west," Dr. Torrey instructed me. The State of California, and Los Angeles in particular, is the epicenter of the catastrophe. The state has been "the canary in the coal mine from day one," he said, because it emptied out its hospitals early. In 1975, the city's "containment" policy squeezed people with substance abuse disorders, mental illness, and other disabilities into a fifty-block radius—skid row—helping it become what a *Los Angeles Times* reporter called "a dumping ground for hospitals, prisons, and other cities to get rid of people with nowhere else to go."[43] Today, roughly fifteen thousand people struggling with serious mental illness live on the streets in Los Angeles,[44] and the Los Angeles County Jail is the largest mental treatment facility in the nation. For many patients needing psychiatric care in the area, the last refuge is the busiest emergency room in America at LAC+USC Medical Center.

Torrey convinced me that Los Angeles was the place to uncover this story. Before I'd attended Cornell Medical Center in Manhattan in 1988, I started my psychiatry residency at UCLA. From 1987 to 1988, I had trained at UCLA's research and treatment hospital, the Neuropsychiatric Institute. Yet, while in Los Angeles, I'd never set foot into what we, the UCLA residents, referred to as *County*, now called LAC+USC Medical Center. The UCLA

residents kept to the west side of Los Angeles for our training, cush-
ioned by Beverly Hills to the east and the beaches of Santa Monica
to the west. County was downtown where the USC residents
trained, facing desperate people with debilitating mental illnesses
in one of the busiest psych EDs in America.

In the fall of 2012, I walked through its doors for the first time.

CHAPTER 2

ME-TOO MEDICINES

"The truth will set me free. Budabudapup! Namaste. Someone told me that. Someone who was raped told me that. Budabudapup! I love everybody. Who drives the van? I don't know. My truth will set me free. Am I house of spirit? Am I *Sophie's Choice*? Who will ever know? . . . Budabudapup! Reboot!"

Johanna's words come out rapid-fire, punctuated by the cartoonish robot noise she repeats over and over. Wearing a NASA shirt and a clear plastic bag tied around her entire body below the neck, the young white woman with cropped reddish-brown hair and freckles sits in a waiting area of the psychiatric emergency department of LAC+USC Medical Center, one of the largest and busiest public hospitals in the United States. When the police ask her if they can take off the handcuffs (that she had requested they put on her), she refuses. "Nope. Not right now."

A first-year psychiatry resident begins the intake. "All right, Johanna, did you take any drugs today?"

"No. I have too much energy," she replies, kicking her legs in the chair, arms still handcuffed behind her back. "Budabudapup! I saw Michael Jackson die. Budabudapup! I am not who I am. Do you understand? When you look at your shit you will know. Rihanna, you are not the truth, and neither is Oprah for being O."

"Have you ever been on medication before?"

"Lots."

"What kind?"

"Every single one prescribed by my doctor. *The. Rapist.* What does that stand for? Therapist. Spell that out."

The doctor asks if Johanna wants medication to calm her down, but it isn't really a choice. As ED staff holds her arm to give her an injection, she yells, "Nope. Get the fuck out of here! No, no, no. I don't trust. I refuse—get the fuck off of me!"

Johanna gets "the usual" for agitated patients, informally called "the cocktail": a dose of Ativan, a benzodiazepine to calm her to sleep, and an antipsychotic to stop the delusions and hallucinations. Johanna needs a break from her illness, and the cocktail will quickly do the job. It will also help the doctors do their jobs. With the psych ED running at as much as 200 percent of intended capacity, the best patient is one who is calm, cooperative, perhaps even asleep.

Johanna has bipolar disorder with episodes of mania and depression. Today, she is in a manic phase, unable to shut down the engine of her racing mind. Sleep is difficult to impossible. The cocktail calms her, as intended, and staffers roll her in a gurney to a spot against the wall where she sleeps alongside other patients.

My first good look at the psychiatric emergency department at LAC+USC came in October 2012. I had been exposed to similar EDs, but none that compared to this six-hundred-bed teaching facility with thousands of employees, connected to the highly regarded Keck School of Medicine at the University of Southern California.

Located in a lower-income, predominantly Latino community called Boyle Heights in downtown Los Angeles, an eight-minute drive southwest to skid row and a six-minute drive west to the county jail, the hospital serves rich and poor, students and homeless people, those with insurance and those without. Once operating out of the Art Deco building dubbed the "Great Stone Mother" that was featured in the opening credits of *General Hospital*, the current medical center is a 1.5-million-square-foot complex of three linked towers, organized around a campus complete with pedestrian plazas and gardens.[1] The emergency department takes up the lion's share of space, and to the right of the emergency entrance, through a set of locked doors managed by an attendant, one enters the world of twenty-first-century emergency psychiatry.

The first time I set foot inside a psychiatric emergency room was in 1980, during my second year at medical school in New York City. My job was to shadow Dr. Calib, a brilliant psychiatric resident who worked the night shift at Bronx Lebanon Hospital. Before we even shook hands, Dr. Calib asked if I was hungry. "Not really," I answered. "Well, here's the thing," he said, "when you're in an emergency room, if there's ever a chance for you to eat, you eat." We got Chinese takeout from a place under the elevated train, during what indeed turned out to be our only opportunity for dinner. When we returned, I was quickly surrounded by insanity like I hadn't seen since I'd lived with Merle. One patient, who was tied to a gurney, managed to free one hand and reach a shelf of vials, pills, and equipment, sweeping it all to the floor. Another patient had set his apartment building on fire. "I like to see the flames," he explained. A half-dozen other consults kept us running from room to room.

At eleven o'clock, Dr. Calib "signed out," downloading information to the incoming psychiatrist as part of the shift change. He mentioned the patient's "I like to see the flames" comment. Hearing Calib relate the patient's absurd explanation caused some floodgate to burst open, and I had to excuse myself. Out in the hallway, behind the closed door, I burst into uncontrollable, horror-stricken, nervous laughter. I couldn't understand how the residents kept it so cool. I finally composed myself, went back in, and apologized. "He's okay," Dr. Calib said to his colleague. "First night."

But nothing would discourage me from becoming a shrink. No other profession seemed remotely possible. No other field held any appeal.

During those years in med school, I had no interest in the microscope. I loathed the cadaver and gave up meat for a year to avoid being reminded of *him* at mealtime. I hated killing the dog to study how the heart stopped. I was bored by the forays to the hospital to do "cool" procedures like inserting a central line into the internal jugular vein. Instead, I started making documentary films about patients with schizophrenia. I took courses at nearby film schools, to connect me to what I loved doing—talking to and trying to understand people like Merle. My parents, who had never liked my choice of specialty, didn't know what to make of me. "If you want to make films, maybe you should become a radiologist?" my mother suggested.

For my psych residency, I moved to Los Angeles for what struck me as the nation's best training, at the University of California Los Angeles (UCLA) Neuropsychiatric Institute. There, working at one of the largest Veterans Administration (VA) hospitals in the country, I began to understand more deeply the complexities of treating SMI thanks to my first teacher, psychiatrist Theodore van Putten,

MD. Dr. van Putten was a fastidious and impeccably dressed man with wire-rimmed glasses and a bow tie. I studied him as much as I did the patients. During early-morning rounds, when patients lined up to talk with him, he would ask, "What's your problem?" After a minute of listening to their complaints, he would dictate their medicine changes to the nurse, then snap, "Next." (I witnessed one patient with schizophrenia throw a trash can after rounds because he felt so disregarded.) Then there was Dr. van Putten's practice of drawing straws. In the 1980s, many people who had taken antipsychotic medicines for decades developed a neurological condition called tardive dyskinesia, characterized by disabling, disfiguring, and irreversible movements of the tongue, arms, and feet. As part of his research on reducing medication quantity to determine the minimum effective dosage and cut down on side effects, Dr. van Putten would have the residents literally draw straws to determine what dosage he'd dole out to each patient who agreed to be part of his research program. The shorter the straw, the lower the dose. Dr. van Putten took careful notes of the results. This randomized research changed the course of prescribing antipsychotic meds: less can be more. He discovered that lower doses often got people better than higher doses, with fewer side effects.

One day I saw him picking trash off the floor, tidying up the hallways for the patients and the visitors, and realized that despite his bullish demeanor, Dr. van Putten cared deeply about his ward and its patients. He wasn't a bleeding heart like most of my other liberal mentors, but unlike all my previous teachers, he was giving blood every day. He was the very first doctor I had ever met who'd dedicated his entire professional life to working in the trenches with the patients who needed him the most: those with schizophrenia. He didn't have a fancy office, just a back room in the VA where he treated patients, day in and day out. The work he did was transformative, launching a legacy of schizophrenia research in Los Angeles and improving the prescribing of antipsychotic meds for millions of people.

Still, I always wondered how this brilliant, dapper, sophisticated man with a taste for the finer things in life ended up spending his days treating the sickest people in a corner of the VA hospital until his death in 1993. Not until I spoke to his protégé and his widow for this book did I learn that Dr. van Putten had a sister with schizophrenia.

• • •

Almost thirty years later, Dr. McGhee, a doctor in the LAC+USC psych ED, is trying to teach her residents how to make the right decisions for the right reasons when prescribing antipsychotic meds. The young resident caring for Johanna tells her: "She's presenting with lack of sleep, distractibility, grandiosity, most recent episode: manic."

Bipolar disorder is diagnosed based on a cluster of symptoms developed by psychiatrists in the twentieth century, among them the frenzied, erratic, tangential speech with a constantly shifting focus that Johanna displays, which psychiatrists call "pressured speech." Other symptoms include periods of marked, elevated, expansive, and grandiose moods with boundless, irrational exuberance and confidence. With mania or hypomania (a less extreme form), people experience periods of euphoria, high energy, sleeplessness, or unusual irritability.

Interspersed with periods of elevated moods are the normal or *euthymic* moods that affect some people with bipolar disorder, along with the plummet of depression. The depression side of the disorder leaves people feeling low and hopeless, often paralyzed by a sense of defeat, blinding pessimism, and fatalism. It also often includes distractibility, slowed thought (so much so that it may be confused with dementia in the elderly), lack of energy, and a loss of interest in the joys in life, including a shutting down of the person's drives for sex, joy, love, health, and food. Bipolar disease can exist with or without losing touch with reality, aka psychosis.

"What do you want to start her on?" asks Dr. McGhee.

"I was thinking Seroquel maybe," says the resident.

"Because . . ." prompts the attending.

"Because at the APA conference they had a study that showed that Seroquel as a stand-alone medication seemed to work very well for the bipolar patients."

The attending prods for more information. "If you would like to start her on Seroquel, that's fine. What would be the downside?"

"It could cause hypotension."

"It's going to be *very* sedating. Some people—boom!—they're on the floor with it. And some people not. I don't know with her. It's going to be a guess."

"You want to know what I learned from the drug rep people?" asks the resident, referring to pharmaceutical representatives who hosted the seminar she attended at the APA's annual meeting.

"Okay, yes."

"They said to start on, for people who are manic, start with like two hundred on the first day, and then increase to, like . . . They said increase gradually so on the fourth day you're on six hundred."

"Think about what their incentive is," cautions Dr. McGhee, "versus what we need to do for the patient." McGhee waits for a nod and then continues her Socratic lesson: "What are the major side effects of Seroquel?"

"Metabolic effects."

"Yes, and Seroquel is *super* high on that."

"And she's, like, a young lady—"

"She's a young lady. We don't necessarily want to fatten her up, but also, we're not necessarily deciding on her long-term meds. But it's important to be aware. That's all I'm saying. Those are some of the conversations you can have in your head about why this versus that one versus the other one."

Johanna is just one of ten million Americans diagnosed with psychotic disorders who need expanded medication options. Richard Friedman, MD, director of psychopharmacology at the Payne Whitney Psychiatric Clinic, tells me that "fifty percent of people at the end of a year stop their treatments, either because the drugs don't make them feel better or they can't tolerate their side effects." Make no mistake about it. On balance, these medicines save lives and are essential for most people to get better. But they are also undoubtedly problematic. According to the Substance Abuse and Mental Health Services Administration (SAMHSA), up to 83 percent of people with SMI are overweight or obese.[2]

The resulting sedation and low self-esteem makes people eat even more, compounding their risk for diabetes and heart disease. They experience a disproportionate number of early deaths, with a reduction in life expectancy of up to twenty-five years, partly as a consequence of type 2 diabetes and cardiovascular disease.[3]

Seroquel, the trade name for quetiapine, is among the atypical, or second-generation, antipsychotic agents marketed in the late 1990s after the release of clozapine broke the "new medication barrier."[4] In Europe in the late 1950s, researchers discovered that clozapine functioned effectively as an antipsychotic *without* causing one of the dreaded and sometimes fatal side effects of existing (first-generation) antipsychotics: a medication-induced fever and delirium called neuroleptic malignant syndrome. Before clozapine, doctors had relied on traditional drugs such as chlorpromazine, the first blockbuster antipsychotic,[5] or haloperidol (brand name Haldol), a chlorpromazine analogue released in 1958.[6] Although these earlier drugs did bring about symptom improvements that allowed many patients to leave institutions, treatment in 40 percent of patients came at the high cost of debilitating and permanent side effects, like extrapyramidal syndrome (EPS), which is characterized by Parkinsonian-like movement disorders.

Enter the second-generation antipsychotics—clozapine, olanzapine, quetiapine, and risperidone—currently used to treat schizophrenia, bipolar disorder, major depressive disorder, and schizoaffective disorder. They were first marketed in the late 1980s and 1990s as being comparably effective as traditional antipsychotics without causing movement disorders.[7] Research has confirmed that these medications can also work for the mania of bipolar disorder.[8] They also have the potential to cause extreme weight gain, diabetes, and some of the same debilitating movement disorder side effects as the older drugs.

Steven Hyman, MD, one of America's most distinguished research psychiatrists, recalls when he entered the field in the 1980s: "It was quite clear that the vast majority of patients with serious psychiatric illness were at best only partially helped by all of the existing treatments." Like many psychiatrists, he was hopeful that a sea change was coming. During Dr. Hyman's tenure as director of NIMH from 1996 to 2001, he oversaw the comparison of old versus new drugs, finding that "tragically, the second-generation antipsychotic drugs other than clozapine [a drug we'll discuss further in the coming pages] were not all that much better." In fact, the newer antipsychotics cause *more* weight gain than the older options.[9]

Now, four decades into his medical career, Dr. Hyman serves as director of psychiatric research at the Broad Institute of MIT and Harvard. He laments that none of the promise of new, better drugs has been realized, and that the diagnostic system of the twentieth century "turned out to also be a mirage—so fundamentally flawed that it actually probably served to impede research" by making it confusing for scientists to study the diseases based on such inaccurate clustering.

• • •

A year after her stay in the LAC+USC psych ED, I visit Johanna in the single-story, pale yellow house where she lives with her dad. Their backyard is a green oasis. Behind the picnic table covered in bright flowerpots, her dad keeps painted lady and monarch butterflies in a screened-in porch, and as we chat Johanna carefully tears open a series of wax-paper envelopes, releasing the colorful insects one by one. The topic quickly turns to meds. She's been hospitalized ten times in the past year but has recently stopped taking the mood stabilizer and antipsychotic drugs she's been prescribed. "So, it's been about three or four months and I find that I, personally, function better off medications."

"I think your mom felt really strongly that you take your medication," says her dad, a cheerful, middle-aged man with white hair and dark eyebrows. "I just wanted to be sure what was the right thing for you. We don't know the side effects that they give you."

Johanna tries to explain. "I didn't say, like, 'I'm not going to take medication. I don't need it.' It was, 'Okay, the medications are making me worse, so let's try it without it.' I mean it's very weird to go into a hospital and then the pills have the opposite effect. Everyone's different. Every *body*, every *person* is going to have different reactions. I wish it was that simple for me. Like, 'Ah! You know, I found this pill and it worked.'"

Johanna, now twenty-three, has been hospitalized more than a dozen times since her first manic episode at age nineteen. Her treatments have included multiple medications aimed at staving off more manic episodes. The cycle of antipsychotic drugs and untreated mania that she describes illustrates the dilemma facing many people with SMI. "When I start to have my mental break, my mind starts to feel like it's turning to mush," she says. "You know how, like, when you see apples or like a pear or something, and they're rotting and they're mushy and they sink in? That's how I feel. That's how my brain feels." As the episode sets in, she stops being able to function normally. "I'm talking really fast, and I can barely sit still, and . . . and getting manic."

But the medications often make her feel worse. "For me, it feels like with each new pill you get a whole new version of craziness." Johanna describes the shift from "talking and screaming and feeling like I have all this energy" to "going really slow," to the point that she can't talk and winds up stuttering, just trying to get the words out.

Those are just the mental side effects. While taking the antipsychotic medication risperidone, Johanna experienced a choking sensation that would come and go. "My neck would stiffen, and I was like, 'Why am I trying to kill myself? Why is my body literally trying to kill itself? I cannot breathe; I'm choking.'" And then she began lactating—a relatively uncommon but known side effect of risperidone, which can disrupt the reproductive endocrine function in women, sometimes raising the hormone prolactin that triggers the breasts to produce milk. And that is "not a benign issue," Lee S. Cohen, MD, director of the Center for Women's Mental Health at Massachusetts General Hospital and professor of psychiatry at Harvard Medical School, tells me. On the contrary, by "turning off reproductive endocrine function and estrogen, [the drug-induced prolactin increase] puts women at risk for early onset of osteoporosis and a whole host of other problems."

But avoiding her meds is also not working in Johanna's favor. Six months after my first visit to her house, she's in trouble and has called for a ride to the hospital. Her father had gotten sick and could no longer live at home. Johanna comes to the door in a boisterous mood, carrying a '76 American flag on a metal pole with an eagle on the top and wearing bright pink lipstick, sparkling gold eye shadow, and a red bandana. Her face and chest are marked up with black and red doodles made in marker or lipstick: stars, hearts, a hash mark, the word *Respect* written in reverse just below her collarbones.

"It's a mess." Johanna sweeps her arm in the direction of the living room behind her. "This is about to get bad," she says with a strained laugh. "But that's how things get better . . . so . . ." Inside, the house is littered with bags, boxes, food, a half-empty water bottle, a set of golf clubs. Towels and clothing, piled high, sit alongside cardboard boxes, some taped and labeled, others open and spilling over.

"Trying to clean it," Johanna explains. "And I made it worse because I'm like, 'You know what I'm going to do? Just take it all out and then we have to deal with it.' And now I can't deal with it." She laughs, but it doesn't hide a flash of despair in her eyes before she shifts back into tour guide mode, pointing out landmarks in the terrain of her turmoil. Her NASA shirt hangs down her back like a cape and a plastic bag is tied around her arm. At breakneck speed, she says, "It's been bad, but it's been good because you have to have the bad times to recognize the good times. The light to rise, wake up! The darkness to slow down, regrow, to up, down, up, die, live, bipolar. I think we all are and it's a blessing, it's a curse and a blessing. It's yin and yang." Demonstrating the rapid cascade of loosely connected ideas that can come with mania, Johanna says, "There's a Japanese art form where when something cracks you fill it in with gold and it becomes better, stronger, faster—Kanye West— the robots."

Passing through the kitchen, which is strewn with dishes, cans and bottles, coffeemakers, cleaning products, and a half-eaten pizza, Johanna describes her latest regimen: "Water, then orange juice, melatonin—so not Xanax or anything like that. Can't do antidepressants, even when I get depressed. Then I try to go more vitamin C, oranges, sunlight." Raw meat sits atop a platter on the windowsill. "Look at this nasty food: this pizza from last night, which I still haven't eaten. I can't even feed myself." She flaps her arms like wings. "I don't know why. This is why I can't get better. Antidepressants that are supposed . . . they crack, triggered the bipolar, which becomes amped-up psycho and makes it worse. I need to sleep," she concludes. "I don't know the last time I've slept."

Johanna packs her bags and slings them over her shoulder. In the car en route to LAC+USC's psych ED, fifty miles away, she explains how she's lost her job. Her boss kept calling to give her shifts but she eventually stopped returning the calls or showing up. Then she didn't have money to pay her phone bill. She scrunches her face, holding back tears. "I'm trying to, like, go to school, and shit keeps knocking me fucking back. Everything that's supposed to get me ahead is knocking me back."

Reaching LAC+USC at last, walking across the hospital's pedestrian bridge, Johanna seems relieved. "It's motherfucking nappy time." No doubt the doctors will offer her the "cocktail" that will help her sleep, but, as always, her relief will only be temporary.

• • •

"The brain does not give up its secrets easily," says Dr. Friedman. This presents significant obstacles to the discovery of new mechanisms for treating mental illness. Because researchers have struggled to identify new molecular targets, individuals with SMI—as well as the doctors who treat them—are left to make do with "me-too" drugs. It takes billions of dollars to develop effective medications with fewer side effects, and the failures of multiple expensive studies have led the pharmaceutical industry to pull back on neuropsych research altogether. "A number of very large drug companies have withdrawn from looking for new treatments for psychotic illness, which is very, very consequential for the field," says Stephen Marder, MD, professor and director of the section on psychosis at the Semel Institute for Neuroscience at UCLA. As a result, there "hasn't been a blockbuster drug in psychiatry for decades."

Without research that might identify novel molecular targets in the brain, many pharmaceutical companies are left to work with the same compounds discovered in the 1950s and 1960s, tweaking them to work slightly better or marginally reduce side effects. The business model is, as Dr. Friedman explains, to make as much profit as possible before their patents run out (which can happen quickly given that the clock starts ticking when the drug is created, *before* it undergoes years of testing and then is brought to the marketplace). As a result, today's antipsychotic and bipolar medications are much safer, are more tolerable, and have fewer side effects, yet they are no more effective in eradicating symptoms, and we are no closer to a cure. Dr. Friedman explains it this way: "The risk-averse pharmaceutical industry takes a known compound with a known mechanism of action and modifies it just slightly to get a 'new drug.' So, you have lots and lots of what we call 'me-too' drugs that are new, they're patented, but they work on exactly the same targets as the old drugs."

In *Scientific American*, Edmund S. Higgins, clinical associate professor of psychiatry and family medicine at the Medical University of South Carolina, offers this analysis:

> As it turns out, drugs developed in the past twenty years perform like older medications. Abilify is no more effective for treating schizophrenia than the very first antipsychotic, Thorazine. New antidepressants lift mood no better than the tricyclic antidepressants discovered in the 1950s. Lithium, first used in 1949, remains the gold standard for bipolar disorder. Adderall provides no further advantages for attention-deficit/hyperactivity disorder than the Benzedrine first administered for it in 1937.[10]

Over the course of my career, I have seen better medications and greater access to care for many patients. But innovation is lacking. As a society, Dr. Friedman explains, we have decided to leave most of the research, development, and testing of medications to the for-profit pharmaceutical industry, rather than to NIMH or other government agencies. Since the brain is so hard to understand and so hard to study, we need much more investment aimed at identifying the basic mechanisms and circuits involved in psychiatric illness. But "that is not something the drug companies are going to spend their money or their time doing," he cautions, laying out the scope of our predicament:

> We don't need fifteen SSRI antidepressants. We don't need twelve new atypical antipsychotics all doing the same thing. What we need are new drugs that act in different systems and different chemicals in the brain and different circuits. That's the crux of the problem in discovering new drugs for psychiatric disorders because in order to do that, you need basic science understanding of psychiatric illness. . . . That's something that basic science researchers in universities are going to do, make discoveries that are interesting about the targets for psychiatric disorders, identify targets, synthesize new drugs, and go to the drug companies and say, "Guess what, we found a fascinating new target. We understand something about schizophrenia or depression that we didn't before, and now we want to partner with you and we want you to go ahead and make and test this."

• • •

One researcher who is working to advance our knowledge as a means of improving care and treatments for people with SMI is

Lisa Dixon, MD, MPH, an internationally recognized scientist and clinician who has received more than twenty-five years of continuous funding from NIMH as well as the VA. Her studies have focused on advancing treatment engagement and adherence, improving quality of care, and reducing the negative impacts of co-occurring substance abuse addictions.

I first met Dr. Dixon in 1988 when I was a third-year resident unpacking boxes in my new office at the New York Hospital–Cornell University Medical Center (NYH-CUMC) after my transfer from UCLA. She was a year ahead of me. After making our introductions, she said, "We have something in common. We both have a sibling with schizophrenia." I stopped short. Someone had divulged the confidential information that I'd disclosed only in my interview—a secret I rarely shared with anyone, much less my colleagues. I must've turned white.

"I guess I said the wrong thing," she said, apologizing. *Shit*, I thought, *my secret is out.* I couldn't stop that. But to make the breach feel less real, I avoided Lisa. We didn't exchange another word for more than thirty years, when I reached out to her for this book.

Dr. Dixon is among the world's leading psychiatrists for people with SMI. A professor of psychiatry at Columbia University Medical Center and director of the Division of Behavioral Health Services and Policy Research, she also serves as editor in chief of *Psychiatric Services*, the most important medical journal for daily care of people with SMI. She directs the Center for Practice Innovations (CPI) at the New York State Psychiatric Institute and leads OnTrackNY, an early-intervention program aimed at reducing disability in people experiencing their first episode of psychosis.

Forty years ago, her brother developed schizophrenia. According to their mother, Jacqueline, Sam had been a sweet, bright child. She noticed the first sign of trouble after he returned from an eight-week bicycle trip in Ireland between high school and college. "When he came back there was an almost imperceptible difference," Jacqueline tells me. "I can't even describe it." Then, after his first term in college, Sam's academics began to decline. He came home every weekend and didn't seem to have made friends at school. He began "doing things in excess," like drinking massive amounts of water or walking the dogs for inordinately long periods of time. "His behavior was not like a normal twenty-year-old," she says, "and we didn't know what to make of it."

At this point Sam still had reasonable social skills, and his symptoms were at a low, manageable level—what is called the *prodrome* or precursor of the fulminating illness. But when he went off to medical school, his behavior grew increasingly disturbed. He never did laundry; he played basketball at odd times of night. He wound up repeating a year, and before long the medical school dismissed him. Jacqueline learned later that his bizarre mannerisms at both college and med school had been widely known to his teachers and peers, but no one had ever informed her or expressed any concern. Had his family known earlier about his decline, she believes they might have been able to help him more quickly. At home, he began having near-physical fights with family members, which was completely out of character. He was drinking eighteen glasses of water a day and became paranoid that the gardener, along with planes overhead, were after him. Then he stopped eating and became catatonic. He was hospitalized for the first time in 1981.

Through helping to manage her brother's treatment, Dr. Dixon quickly learned the value of having a doctor who cares. "He had some hospitalizations. He had some wonderful psychiatrists; he had some psychiatrists who weren't communicative at all. We learned—and I always say this to the psych residents—that the power of a kind, communicative psychiatrist is so much beyond what you could even imagine." Despite her brother's declining condition, her family never gave up. They confronted it head-on, seeking help down every avenue. Dr. Dixon approached the head of mental health services for medical students at the training program where she was a first-year student: John Talbott, MD, who, as luck would have it, was a pioneering advocate for those with SMI. Dr. Talbott worked with Dr. Dixon and her mother, offering them an education that would serve as a model for the type of interventions that Dr. Dixon would come to promote professionally.

Even so, nothing worked. "My brother has a greater severity of illness than probably the average person with schizophrenia," she tells me. He was paranoid and unable to conform to the norms required of him in a group home where, as she explains, "you have to have breakfast when basically everybody else is having breakfast," for example. "My brother didn't like that life." The only possibility was hospitalization—until he started taking an antipsychotic introduced in the United States in the 1980s called clozapine.

The results were transformative. "My brother did very, very well on clozapine; he was out of the hospital, he was functioning," says Dr. Dixon. Although he was still unable to work, "you could talk to him about the basketball game, you could play Ping-Pong. He really just became himself. He became my brother again. He didn't have a job, he didn't get married. None of those things. But he seemed to be happy. He became more like the person I knew, a very gentle, kind of unassuming guy."

Doctors live in fear of their prescriptions resulting in deadly side effects and always want to operate in accordance with the "First, do no harm" promise of the Hippocratic oath. When a blood test result raised concerns that Sam might have developed a potentially fatal side effect, he was taken off the drug. Called agranulocytosis, this side effect of clozapine causes the immune system's white blood cells to shut down. Once Sam was off the drug, his subsequent mental decline was rapid. "He was horrible. He was as sick as I've ever seen him. He was disorganized, paranoid, and had no interest in basketball." After his doctors determined that clozapine was not causing agranulocytosis, Dr. Dixon and his mother convinced them to put him back on the drug that had helped him so much. Unfortunately, as sometimes happens, he never recovered to the same degree. "He just never really was able to rebuild his life after that," Dr. Dixon tells me. To this day, he occupies a long-term bed at one of the nation's few remaining state institutions. Now sixty-one, he is unlikely to ever recover without a major breakthrough in treatment options.

One of the differentiating features of clozapine, first synthesized for psychiatric illness in 1958, sold in Europe in 1972, and finally marketed in the United States in 1990, was its effectiveness for the 30 percent of people with schizophrenia who are "treatment refractory," meaning that they have not responded to three trials of antipsychotic medications from at least two different classes.[11] This meant that clozapine could ease the symptoms of many of the sickest patients whose condition had, before the drug, been only marginally improved, or not at all improved by treatment. It also effectively managed what psychiatrists refer to as the "negative" effects of schizophrenia—cognitive deterioration and social withdrawal—and not just the "positive" symptoms such as hallucinations and delusions. As John Crilly writes in his history of the medicine, clozapine "forced the psychopharmaceutical industry to move forward into the twenty-first century," while also giving "another group of people suffering from severe, treatment-refractory schizophrenia hope for a better quality of life."[12]

I learned more about this transformative drug from Dr. Dixon's husband, Donald Goff, MD, professor of psychiatry at NYU School of Medicine and director of the Nathan Kline Institute for Psychiatric Research. For the twenty-five years before he moved to New York City, Dr. Goff had been director of a community mental health outpatient clinic in Boston associated with Harvard Medical School that was one of the leading centers of its kind. He has studied clozapine for nearly three decades, in both laboratory and clinical settings.

He tells me that for many doctors, prescribing clozapine seems like "too much trouble" because of the monitoring necessary to protect against the agranulocytosis that's estimated to occur in 1 to 2 percent of treated patients.[13] Patients on clozapine require weekly blood tests, and this level of sustained care would be difficult for anyone who isn't in an inpatient setting but is particularly difficult to manage with folks with SMI. Regardless, Dr. Goff says, compared to high-risk cancer treatments, for example, clozapine is relatively safe. And given the remarkable results he's observed, he thinks it should be much more widely prescribed. "A third of all of our patients were on clozapine," he says. "For many of them, it changed their lives. It allowed chronically hospitalized people to be discharged. It allowed people who were chronically suicidal or aggressive to have that under control." Among his several hundred clinic patients taking the drug, roughly half improved, and very few wound up hospitalized, although many still had some psychotic symptoms. "It seems to protect people from relapse and exacerbation. It decreases hospitalizations probably for life," he says.

He is such a believer in the drug that despite the high-stakes side effects, he tells me that "if someone continues to have psychosis with the other antipsychotic drugs, it's bordering on medical malpractice to not offer clozapine."

But Dr. Dixon, who oversees hundreds of providers, understands the dilemma that a drug such as this one creates for doctors in the trenches. Imagine that you're a psychiatrist with a caseload of five hundred or one thousand SMI patients, she says. You don't want patients on a drug that requires such close monitoring, especially when many patients are unreliable about keeping appointments.

To me, it seems remarkable that a drug discovered sixty years ago, which has all this health, administration, and oversight baggage, remains the gold standard for effectiveness. Six decades later, it's equally dumbfounding that we still don't understand *why* clozapine is more effective than other drugs. Given the woeful state of psychopharmaceutical research today, Dr. Friedman rightfully calls for "much more basic science in terms of the basic mechanisms and circuits that are involved in psychiatric illness."

Meanwhile, people like Johanna have to make do with the available treatments. Five years after we first met, Johanna says, "I finally realized that I do have bipolar. You know, a lot of people don't need to be on meds, but unfortunately I'm not one of them." She has also come to recognize that her relapses are part of her disease. Instead of being a reason to stop taking the drugs prescribed to her, it's a sign that it's time to adjust the dosages. And she's doing her best to cope with the significant side effects. "The Zyprexa makes me so hungry. I feel like a bear that has just this never-ending appetite and I just eat big portions," she says. "I think big can be beautiful. But for me, at this size, even standing too long or walking short distances, my back hurts. Even when I go on my walks—when I try to do what it takes to feel better—I feel worse, like my back just hurts so I have to stop a lot." The meds also make it hard for her to focus. "It's like I have ADD. It's hard for me to pick up a book and read, and I'm a huge reader. But it keeps me stable."

Despite having come to accept her condition, Johanna is distressed that she can't really function in the world or be independent. "It's my twenties. I'm supposed to be alive!" She tells me she plans to update her résumé and apply to the dollar store across the street, maybe even return to school. But she worries that anyone who knows about her situation will look down on her. "I feel like someone's gonna be like, 'Oh you're a societal mooch. You mooch off your parents. You mooch off society. You mooch off the school.' And I'm trying so hard. When you saw me the very first time where I'm wearing the trash bag and stuff, I was working two jobs and going to night school. I'd already spent two years at a homeless shelter trying to get work, trying to save up, going to therapy, trying to work, and I couldn't do it." She recognizes how hard it is for others with mental illness who may not have had the same privileges as she has. "I'm college educated. I don't have any [physical] disabilities. I don't have racism going against me. I don't have a violent background. I didn't grow up with parents who beat me or anything," she explains. "If I can't make it, what about everyone else?"

CHAPTER 3

DUNGEONS AND DRAGONS: CRIMINALIZING MENTAL ILLNESS

Monte stands in the doorway of Seclusion Room B, a white sheet tied across his shoulders like a cape, wearing a hospital gown and a neon patient bracelet around each wrist. When a petite white woman in scrubs with cropped hair approaches, Monte, who's African American, straightens up his six-foot-two-inch, 220-pound frame and backs cautiously into the room. "Yes, ma'am," he says, clearly bracing himself even as he towers over her.

Nurse Practitioner Ellis speaks calmly and directly. An acquaintance of Monte's sister, she was asked to come to help smooth Monte's transition into what will be his fifth hospitalization in fifteen years. Now it's time for him to leave the ED. "A couple of things: when they take you to this other place, one, just try to remember it's a hospital."

"If there's no red dragons there," Monte replies, matter-of-fact. "If there's a red dragon there it's all bad because I don't get on with the red dragon."

"Okay," Nurse Ellis responds, equally matter-of-fact. "I don't know if there are or not—"

"Let me stop you right there," Monte interrupts, his expression shifting to confidence and courage. "It really doesn't matter if there is, because if he's there I'll take his ass out anyway. So, it doesn't matter. Okay, go on."

"So, they're going to take you in an ambulance—"

"Okay, let me think about this a second. Ambulance," he ponders. "An ambulance is going at its right rate it should get me there in a certain amount of time, but if somebody tries to intrude and crash over and kidnap me and hold me hostage, then what are you going to do?" He pauses. "See, you've got to be able to answer these questions to make sure your methods work," he challenges, as if the two were speaking in the War Room, strategizing for the next battle.

"They are going to restrain you when you go, so you can just get prepared." At once, Monte recedes into a back corner of the room, rolling his body against the wall.

"Restraint! Restraint!" he repeats over and over.

"I know. It's a pain in the butt," Nurse Ellis says, her voice quiet and calm.

"Restraint. When you say the word *restraint* it's a big trigger. I'll explain something to you real quick. When they say the word *restraint*, okay, it goes like this. One, two—" As Monte yells "RESTRAINT!" he lands in a martial artist's fighting stance, bobbing side to side, never losing eye contact with his invisible opponent.

Nurse Ellis doesn't flinch. "Yeah, I know," she says. "That's why I'm kind of trying to give you a heads-up."

When presenting Monte's case to the chief of the psychiatric emergency department, Nurse Ellis explained that he's been in a psychotic state for days and off his meds for at least several weeks. His family has been trying to care for him at home but reached the limit of what they can provide. Ever since they learned about his illness, they've done their best to protect him. But it took years for his mother, his sister, and the rest of Monte's loved ones to fully understand what was wrong.

In his late teens, Monte began acting strangely. His younger sister, Patrisse, recalls thinking that his wild mood swings and the hours he spent locked in the bathroom sobbing were caused by his smoking crack. Although he was using street drugs to self-medicate, that was only part of the problem.[1] "There were days and nights when my brother did not sleep," she later wrote in her memoir, but instead "chattered on incessantly."[2] At age nineteen, he was arrested while psychotic and charged with attempted robbery. The jail psychiatrist diagnosed him with schizoaffective disorder, which explained his bizarre behaviors. But according to Monte's family, no one shared that information with them. Only years later did they learn that he had been hearing voices at the time of his arrest.

People with schizoaffective disorder typically experience a combination of symptoms of schizophrenia (which can include hallucinations or delusions) and mood disorders (such as mania or depression). The mental disorder comes in varying levels of intensity and dysfunction and manifests differently in different individuals. It is far less understood (and less strictly defined) than other psychiatric diseases.

In Monte's case, his mental illness made his incarceration even more traumatic. Once, when he was in the midst of an episode, the guards did a cell extraction. The guards kept saying, "'Come out your cell. Come out your cell.' And he was too scared," Patrisse explains. "And so, they started tear-gassing him and Mace-ing him. That," she says, "is what you do to enemy combatants, not people who are citizens of your country."

Reporter Alisa Roth, who spent significant time in the Los Angeles County Jail's Twin Towers, where Monte was incarcerated, researching her book *Insane: America's Criminal Treatment of Mental Illness*, describes the process this way:

Deputies "put on protective equipment that is basically riot gear—knee and elbow pads, helmets, and large plastic shields. They may start by releasing pepper spray into the cell to try to encourage the person to 'cuff up' (get handcuffed) and come out. If the person doesn't come out, then the deputies come into the cell, where they use their shields to get the person up against the wall, or onto the floor, where they can restrain him for transport. . . . Even when everything goes right, an extraction is a frightening experience, all the more so for a person who is psychotic and/or paranoid."[3]

When I asked Monte about how he was treated there, he had few words. "It was just horrible, you know? I don't even like talking about it."

Monte's deep-seated fear of hospitals and anyone in a law enforcement uniform is what convinced his support team to do everything they could to keep him at home for as long as possible. When they arrived, he had growled at a security guard. Nurse Ellis told the psych ED chief that they were trying to "keep him away from the deputies." Despite his psychosis and his formidable size, she was not scared of Monte. "I think he's terrified. He's like a little kid. He's wearing this medallion that he's latched on to that he thinks will keep him safe. He really doesn't feel safe."

• • •

Monte's fear and trauma are not just a product of psychosis but a consequence of experience. Mental illness is never easy. It also acts as what New York City's first lady Chirlane McCray calls a "hardship multiplier"—it makes any problem exponentially worse. As the wife of Mayor Bill de Blasio, she seeks to raise up mentally ill people of all races and religions. McCray, who is African American, is keenly aware of what SMI can mean for people of color, and black people especially. She tells me, "You take someone who's a person of color, already there are significant challenges in that person's life—truly significant when it comes to employment, education, where someone can live, all those things—and you throw mental illness in there . . ." Meanwhile, she says, only 5 percent of psychologists in this country are African American (there are even fewer African American psychiatrists). As a consequence, black people are more likely to get care from nonblack providers, which can lead to miscommunication, inaccurate diagnoses, and subpar care.[4] Research shows that mental health professionals are more likely to see a person of color as sicker than a white person with the same clinical presentation.[5] Providers are also more likely to view a person of color as having a poorer prognosis, needing higher doses of medicine, being more dangerous, and belonging in jail (as opposed to a hospital).[6] As William Lawson, MD, PhD, chair of psychiatry at Howard University, told an industry newspaper, "Aberrant behavior is more likely to send them [African Americans] into the criminal justice system, a punitive approach to mental illness."[7]

That, in short, has been Monte's lived experience. For years, his sister has shouldered valid concern about his safety. She braces herself against the terror that her brother will die at the hands of the police, not understanding or unable to follow their commands. Given that roughly a quarter of the people shot by police have a history of mental illness[8] and a vastly disproportionate number of them are African American,[9] Patrisse's fear is not unfounded. Monte has already had at least one close call.

At age twenty-six, he stopped taking his medication regularly. In the midst of a psychotic episode, he got into a minor car accident and when the police arrived, he bolted. They shot him down with rubber bullets. "Next thing, we were visiting him at the hospital," Patrisse recalls. They found him handcuffed to the bedpost. "I could tell he was not well—that he was in an episode." She'd long ago learned to recognize her brother's symptoms: his irritability, erratic sleeping habits, pressured speech, and delusional thoughts.

Their family has assiduously avoided involving the police since 2003. At the time, Monte's mental health had deteriorated significantly, and after EMTs refused to transport him to the hospital once they heard he'd been incarcerated, Patrisse had called the police and made them promise they wouldn't hurt her brother before showing them in. She tried to explain to Monte that they were only there to help. But he dropped to his knees, weeping, his arms in the air. "Please don't take me back. Please don't take me back," he sobbed. She shooed the police away and curled up next to him on the floor.

From that point forward, Monte's friends and family rallied together whenever he was in crisis. "We've made a commitment that whenever he's in an episode we will never call the police," she explains. "We'll just take care of it ourselves. We always have a conversation with him, no matter how present he is or isn't," Patrisse says. "We always say, 'Monte, we're noticing this. We think the hospital might be a good place.'" And then his "front-line team" works together to get him to the emergency room.

Over the years of Monte's cycling in and out of hospitals and jails, Patrisse has kept that promise. She decided after the incident in 2003 that "I was going to be with him, no matter what, and I was going to see him through every episode, and I was going to see him through every downfall and every jail sentence, and everything that was around his mental illness. I was going to make sure that I was way more equipped to deal with it than I felt, like, really, society was. And then I forced all my family to figure it out."

The way that Monte's loved ones have created their own crisis intervention team is impressive on its own, but Patrisse's public work to combat racism has been off the charts. In 2014, she invited me to join her at a vigil outside the Los Angeles Police Department (LAPD) headquarters in memory of Ezell Ford, a twenty-five-year-old black man with mental illness who had been shot dead by LAPD officers in August. On that late-summer day, Ford's name had entered a long and growing list of individuals who have died at the hands of law enforcement and corrections officials—horror stories that have become a feature of the daily news. On a piece of cardboard with a marker, Patrisse wrote out the name of an organization she had just cofounded. She called it Black Lives Matter. What began as a hashtag had become a movement.

Fueled by her fierce love for her brother, Patrisse has become, over the few years I have known her, not only a key advocate of improving conditions for people with mental illness in Los Angeles but also one of the leading civil rights activists in the twenty-first century. "Black Lives Matter really becomes alive inside of me because of the things I witnessed," she explains on the eve of the launch of her memoir. "*Mental illness* has become synonymous with *criminal*. We want to change that, and we want to change the idea of who these folk are. I think if we could change the plight for people with severe mental illness, we could change a lot of things in this country."

Everyone I've followed over the course of my quest has taught me a great deal and inspired me. But it's Patrisse who has pushed me toward activism. Instead of hiding the truth about her family, she has used it as a rallying cry.

• • •

Mental illness crises are the only health emergency in which law enforcement are the first responders. This crystallizing statement from many advocates has opened my eyes to a reality that most of us, including me, have taken for granted. A national survey of law enforcement that tallied the 10 million annual emergency transports for people with mental illness in 2017 found that 70 percent of emergency transports resulted from dispatched calls, with the remainder through unplanned encounters on patrol.[10] While 19 percent of these planned or unplanned encounters were resolved at the scene, the remaining 81 percent required law enforcement to provide transportation to some sort of facility. Of these, 32 percent of the time that was a general hospital emergency department; 22 percent involved transports to a crisis center or psychiatric emergency department. The remaining 27 percent was divided between jail and an inpatient facility, with slightly more transports to jail (15 percent versus 12 percent).

Perhaps most striking of all the survey's findings were tallies of the resources allocated to these transports. *Twenty-one percent of all staff time* for law enforcement officers was spent on mental health transports, which has to do with the fact that they wait an average of three hours for a transfer of custody in a medical facility and an average of thirty-seven minutes in a jail. This work also absorbs a huge amount of money. According to respondents, 10 percent of their overall budget was spent responding to or transporting individuals with mental illness, amounting to a total of $918 billion nationwide.[11] These budgets are funded with taxpayer dollars, revealing our society's significant investment in what is ultimately a failed—and dangerous—approach. As a result, families, seeing no other options, often rely on law enforcement to wrestle their dysfunctional and destructive relatives to a safer place, turning our police departments into the nation's largest psychiatric outreach team.

Over the past several years, police shootings like the one that killed Ezell Ford have received increasing public attention and awareness that it's largely people of color who are the victims—particularly black men and boys. What is less well known is that at least 21 percent of all 992 people who were shot and killed by police in 2018 had a mental illness.[12]

Even once they are brought into custody, people with SMI are in danger. In August 2018, the *Virginian-Pilot* shared stories of 404 people with mental illness who had died in America's jails between 2010 and the summer of 2018.[13] The numbers paint a bleak picture.

- In at least 41 percent of the cases, the individual died in isolation or shortly after being in solitary confinement, which has long been known to exacerbate psychiatric symptoms.

- Forty-four percent of people died by their own hand, alone and unwatched, despite the fact that suicide can often be prevented with regular safety checks and monitoring.

- Seventy individuals died after being restrained, pepper-sprayed, and/or shocked with a stun gun or Taser.

- In at least 11 percent of the cases, family or friends had informed jail officials that their loved one had a mental illness. With six of the victims, someone had tried to bring the correct medications to the jail.

Without proper treatment and medication, people with diagnoses like schizophrenia can decompensate quickly in a jail environment. While *scatolia*, the clinical term for playing with feces, is rarely seen in the outside world, it is a regular occurrence among incarcerated people with SMI,[14] indicating the depths of their dysfunction and desperation.

The dozens of people I've spoken with who work in correctional facilities all admit that treatment of incarcerated individuals is beyond inadequate. America's three largest jails—the Twin Towers in Los Angeles, Chicago's Cook County Jail, and Rikers Island in New York City—serve as the country's three largest psychiatric inpatient facilities. In each county throughout the nation, jails hold more people with mental illness than local inpatient units.[15] Although some renewed attention has come to the problem, it continues to escalate. In the 1970s, about 5 percent of those incarcerated had an SMI. In 2014, 20 percent of inmates in jails and 15 percent of inmates in state prisons did, which translates to approximately 383,000 "individuals with severe psychiatric disease" living behind bars.[16]

Of the approximately sixteen thousand people housed in the Los Angeles County Jail's seven buildings on any given day, about 25 percent of the men and 40 percent of the women need mental health treatment.[17] The challenges that this facility faces—providing proper care for massive numbers of seriously ill individuals while struggling with insufficient resources—are emblematic of jails and prisons across the country.

As part of my journey to document the realities on the ground at the epicenter of the crisis, I sought out the chance to tour Twin

Towers. With the help of then Lieutenant Governor (now Governor) Gavin Newsom, I was allowed into the technologically advanced areas of the facility, where thousands of men in pods live behind Plexiglas under the constant surveillance of cameras monitored by guards perched in elevated posts. We toured what felt like the world's largest fishbowl, or a real-life *Truman Show*, to see the temporary home of thousands of people whom, as Newsom explains, "we've completely given up on." While we sit in front of the Plexiglas, he reminds me that it's not just a California problem and says, "The state mental illness in this country is beyond the trite notion of crisis; it's at a point of comedic absurdity."

The deputy director for community health for the Los Angeles County Department of Health Services—the agency that took over medical care in the county jail system in 2016—Mark Ghaly, MD, MPH, who oversees correctional medicine as well as projects aimed at diverting people with SMI away from incarceration, says, "Emergency rooms are overrun, cops are tired of all the 'wall time' that they have in EDs, so jails become the easiest drop-off place ever. One of my favorite lines—it's not my line, but it's one that made an impression on me early in my work in L.A.—was something one of the advocates said: 'The jail bed is the bed that never says no.'"

I sought similar access at Rikers Island, New York City's main jail complex where, as happens throughout the nation, people with SMI who commit minor crimes often receive major punishments. Many of those at Rikers wind up behind bars after being charged with (although not yet convicted of) small infractions because they're unable to post a couple hundred dollars in bail. In 2011, my requests to film and write about the experiences of people with SMI at Rikers were denied despite staunch support from the city's future mayor, then public advocate, Bill de Blasio. (That refusal made sense to me years later when the *New York Times* released a report of "brutal and routine" violence at the facility.[18] In a single year, 129 inmates had suffered serious injuries—including fractures, wounds requiring stitches, and head injuries—during altercations with staff. In 80 percent of those cases, inmates reported being beaten while handcuffed. Seventy-seven percent had a mental illness diagnosis.)

I was finally permitted to visit and speak with staff in the spring of 2012. Like most New Yorkers, I had no idea where the jail was before I went. Located on a 413-acre island in the East River between Queens and the Bronx, it is just a few blocks away from La Guardia airport. Although it is much larger than the airport, few signs indicate the jail's location. Following the detailed directions that I'd been given by the NYC Department of Corrections (DOC), I turned into a massive parking lot where a DOC official took me over a small bridge that led to another world—a city of concrete jailhouse buildings, surrounded by the glistening East River. The river itself warehoused the overflow of incarcerated people on a converted barge.

After an eight-hour tour of the island, as day gave way to dusk, one of the high-ranking officials drove me around to point out a few more landmarks. After a few minutes, he pulled over, pointed to a building on my right, and spoke, quietly, on the condition of anonymity. "In this building we have situations where mentally ill inmates are disciplined by the other prisoners," he said. When guards decided noncompliance merited punishment, they would leave cell doors ajar so that incarcerated people with SMI deemed "unruly" could be "disciplined" by their peers.

Jails and prisons need order. Many people with SMI find it hard to understand and follow protocols. And their jailers are often at a loss about how to manage them. According to Dr. Torrey, the average stay for all inmates on Rikers Island is 42 days, while the average stay for incarcerated people with mental illness is 215 days—the main reason being that they often cannot understand or follow the rules.[19] All the more reason why activists, advocates, and city officials are determined to close Rikers by 2027 and replace it with smaller, community-based jails throughout the city's five boroughs.

Of all the many issues facing people with SMI—on par with the lack of medical research, the paucity of new treatments, the lack of a national strategy, the enduring stigma, and our disabling shame— criminalization is particularly costly. And that cost is borne by taxpayers. The price of caring for incarcerated people with mental illness far exceeds that of other individuals. In *American Psychosis*, Dr. Torrey outlines a spate of examples that paint the dismal picture:

> In Florida's Broward County jail in 2007, the difference was $130 versus $80 per day. In Texas prisons in 2003, mentally ill prisoners cost $30,000 to $50,000 per year compared to $22,000 for other prisoners. In Washington State prisons in 2009, the most seriously mentally ill prisoners cost $101,653 each, compared to approximately $30,000 per year for other prisoners. And these costs do not include the costs of lawsuits being increasingly brought against county jails, such as the suit brought in New Jersey in 2006 by the family of a sixty-five-year-old mentally ill stockbroker [who was] stomped to death in the Camden County jail.[20]

By shifting the burden of care from hospitals to overcrowded jails, we have re-created the dysfunctional, abusive dynamic that once plagued the institutions deemed so inhumane that they needed to be shut down in the 1960s. Fortunately, new efforts to divert people with SMI from incarceration are springing up nationwide. One sunny spot on the map is Miami-Dade County, Florida, where Judge Steve Leifman, associate administrative judge in the county court's Criminal Division, and chair of the Eleventh Judicial Circuit's Mental Health Committee, walked me through the recent changes that have vastly reduced the jail population, shifting tens of thousands of people out of the criminal justice system. Judge Leifman tells me that in the last eight-plus years, more than six thousand police officers in the City of Miami and Miami-Dade County Police Departments as well as all the city and county's 911 dispatchers have participated in crisis intervention team (CIT) training. Each department or substation in the county has a liaison officer who meets on a quarterly basis with a coordinator and the program's mental health providers. This, he says, "has been wonderfully enabling for the police officers to be able to identify people that are falling through the cracks—bringing them to the attention of the provider authority, to make sure that these individuals are getting the attention they need."

Since the program was implemented, the city and county police departments have handled 83,427 mental health calls, which resulted in a mere 149 arrests, according to Judge Leifman. "Our jail audit was cut almost in half." By keeping most people with SMI from entering the criminal justice system in the first place, "we closed one of our main jails." Not only that, he continued, "we have seen a massive, massive reduction in the number of arrests. We're seeing a massive reduction in the number of police shootings, a massive reduction in police injuries, and a massive reduction in injuries to people with mental illness."

Today, communities nationwide are making similar efforts to reduce the numbers of encounters between people with SMI and law enforcement—or at least to ensure that when police are called the responding officers have received some training in coping with SMI crises. Although they are not yet widespread, CITs operate in nearly 2,700 American communities, according to the University of Memphis CIT Center, which started CIT and offers on its website a national map with instructions on how to find the closest available CIT.[21]

Back in New York City, McCray is working to reduce the need for law enforcement officials to serve as first responders. Her program, ThriveNYC, will spend $850 million over four years to provide a full array of municipal programs to address mental illness in NYC[22]: establishing mobile CITs; diverting people with mental illness out of jail and into treatment; providing mental health prevention and intervention programs in public spaces such as schools, shelters, and senior citizen centers; violence prevention training; the training of community-based mental health providers; and dozens of other services. One of the programs is what is known as "mental health first aid," which in NYC means a free eight-hour training for 250,000 New Yorkers. Like CPR for mental health, it helps people "recognize the early signs and symptoms of mental illness and substance misuse," "learn how to listen without judgment," manage a crisis, and assist people in psychiatric distress until they can connect with professional care. It is all part of her broader initiative to educate about and destigmatize SMI.[23]

For McCray, these issues hit "very close to home." Her daughter,

Chiara, has been forthright in the press about her struggles with depression and addiction, and McCray's own parents were clinically depressed. She also experienced trauma borne of growing up in a white community in the 1950s and 1960s, but "there was little discussion about it" in her family.

Although efforts like McCray's are a critical step in the right direction, the fact remains that, whether we like it or not, police remain our first responders for most mental health crises, and the criminal justice system is the decisive arbiter in the care of individuals with SMI. Today, if you are an American with mental illness, you are up to ten times more likely to be incarcerated than hospitalized.[24] People who work in law enforcement never asked to become our nation's mental health providers. One sheriff of a large city system on the east coast summed up his thankless job this way: "You give us [people you treat like] your trash and then you blame us for mishandling them." In America, people like my sister have become throwaway people.

CHAPTER 4

THROWAWAY PEOPLE

"I'm coming for you," barks Todd. Minutes earlier, he was sitting in the psych ED waiting area. A middle-aged white man with a crew cut, reading a newspaper with glasses perched on the end of his nose, he would hardly have looked out of place in my corner diner on Manhattan's Upper East Side. But his calm demeanor didn't last long.

Concerned for his well-being after seeing him earlier that day, his psychiatrist at the LAC+USC outpatient clinic had sent him to the emergency room. Now Todd seemed hell-bent on provoking nearly everyone, yelling at doctors to get him the correct meds and ordering the nurse who asked him to change out of his clothes to get him some pants—"man's pants" because "I'm not a girl." Todd, forty-seven, had spent more than twenty years behind bars, and now lives on the streets of Los Angeles.

During his intake, he was given two hospital wristbands. When a nurse approaches with scissors to cut off one of the bracelets, Todd jerks his arm away aggressively enough that security officers begin flooding the area. He shouts at the nurse for "coming at" him. An officer asks him to stand and Todd knows exactly what's coming next. He throws down the newspaper with a "*FUCK!*" and puts his hands behind his back, the movements practiced and familiar. The officer handcuffs him, then asks him to sit back down. "Just help us out, for my safety and your safety," he says calmly, patting Todd on his back and directing him toward the chair.

Admitting psychiatrist Dr. McGhee approaches. "What just happened?"

Todd begins to rail. "What happened is these motherfuckers have been fucking with me for over twenty years." His anger quickly pivots in her direction once she tells him she wants him to "hang out in a seclusion room for a while." No handcuffs, she reassures him, "but the door will be locked."

"So now you wanna put me in another cell," he says. "This is what I fucking get every fucking time." He stands, taunting the four sheriff's deputies who guide him away. "Come on, you dick-ass cops! You punk-ass motherfuckers. I come to a fucking hospital, man, and I get treated like I'm back in fucking prison." Dr. McGhee apologizes, saying that isn't her intention.

When I ask her a short time later what makes people turn hostile so quickly, she says, "It was brewing already." Because she had spoken with Todd's clinic doctor before he arrived, she had a sense of what was coming. Todd has bipolar disorder and is in the midst of a "mixed mania" episode—a combination of depressive and manic symptoms. His doctor worried about what he might do to himself. For some people, mania doesn't manifest as energetic happiness but as irritability—an "angry kind of driven emotion, lots of energy, no sleep for days, which is what he's in the middle of," as Dr. McGhee describes it. He may have been abused in jail, Dr. McGhee says, his traumatic memories triggered by the handcuffs and the seclusion room. All that "emotion and energy biologically driven by the underlying disease and the personality characteristics on top of it is a deadly combination."

Then Dr. McGhee admits something. "I really love psychosis," she says. "It's a strange thing to say, but . . . what makes this job interesting is when people are not entirely connected with reality." Still, that disconnect adds significant challenges to her efforts. "The number one obstacle for treating people with mental illness is that they [sometimes] have no insight," she continues, "no ability to be objective about their own behavior and what's going on. It's like *Alice in Wonderland: Through the Looking Glass.* Everything is sort of warped."

The experience of not knowing you're psychotic is part and parcel of SMI. It has a medical name, anosognosia, the inability to see an illness in ourselves that is painfully evident to those around us. Many of us are in denial about our flaws, but not knowing you're psychotic has epic consequences, from inhibiting patients' cooperation with treatment to leading them to barrel full-steam-ahead on irrational, often perilous journeys. Instead of displaying the instinct for self-preservation that carries most of us through life, people in the throes of SMI with anosognosia often seem to be on a quest for destruction.

By this point I'm not surprised to hear that Dr. McGhee's perspective is personal as well as professional. Just after she graduated from medical school, her brother was hospitalized and diagnosed with bi-polar disorder. "Taking my brother to the hospital was the hardest thing I ever had to do," she recalls. She had to educate her family about her sibling's illness. It later propelled her into her job in ED psychiatry. With a sly smile, Dr. McGhee tells me that since most psychiatrists hate the ED, supply and demand means she is fortunate to have a relatively high-paying job that her colleagues avoid. When she was first hired, that salary allowed her to help pay for her broth-er's uncovered medical expenses and his college tuition.

Minutes earlier, when Dr. McGhee wrote up the orders for

medication, she called for pills that Todd agreed to take before he was handcuffed. Now she considers giving him a shot instead. Injecting the drugs into the muscles of the shoulder or buttocks would get them into the bloodstream—and therefore the brain—faster than pills, but she wants to avoid causing even incidental pain to a man who is already so agitated.

Then, in the midst of her paperwork, a scuffle in the hallway outside the seclusion room draws her back to the area. The door that the doctor ordered locked was never locked, and Todd has re-emerged. The security officers ask him to return to the room.

"You guys are gonna lock me in there? You know what's gonna happen when I come out of there, it's gonna be a cell extraction. I'm gonna come for *her*," he seethes. "I'm letting you know that right now." Todd turns toward his doctor. "I'm coming for you!" he yells, walking toward Dr. McGhee. A nurse ushers her away as officers surround Todd.

"Code green. Code green," a nurse calls out, her voice pinched. "Push the panic button!" With that, the hospital announcement system summons the crisis management team. As the officers struggle with Todd, a staffer arrives with a green nylon bag. Todd screams as police and security staff pin him to a table. They wrap a white sheet around his head to prevent him from biting or spitting, which would pose additional risk given his HIV-positive status.

The tight fabric outlines the contours of Todd's anguished face and a red stain emerges in the left corner of his mouth: a small line of blood is spreading toward his ear. Officers call for a spit mask—a hood made of thin, breathable fabric that will replace the sheet. Dr. McGhee stands at a distance, shaking her head. Todd lies spread-eagle and hooded, secured to the table with wide leather straps around his wrists and ankles.

I watch the Code Green team as they emerge from the room, with a sense of accomplishment as the nurse thanks the deputies with "Good call, officer." Everyone recognizes that their "victory" over Todd is a Pyrrhic one. No one more than Dr. McGhee. Her half smile belies an awareness of the futility of this victory over an impaired man that might just lead her to tears.

In that moment, I flash on memories of Merle struggling with my parents. As a child, I often watched my family act out a horrific choreography over and over again. Weary from her school day, Merle would lash out at my mother, threatening and sometimes hitting her until my mother called my father home from work. When he arrived, Merle would shift her attention, taunting him with profanities, calling him names and then retreating to the bathroom and locking the door. Only a deeply troubled fifteen-year-old girl would start a fight with a man like my dad—a former boxer with legendary strength. The scene would inevitably end with the bathroom door broken open, my father's belt in his hands, and my sister in the porcelain tub. He never hit her, to the best of my knowledge, but the belt served to intimidate and subdue her. Once Merle was no longer combative, my mother would rush to her aid, turn on my father, and call him a brute. My dad would leave in a huff. On more than one occasion, he threatened divorce.

The incident with Todd also reminds me of hearing Merle get dragged through the doors of the mental hospital for her second hospitalization, after I'd driven her there under the false pretense of a regular doctor's appointment. I recall her cries for help when they pulled her through the doors—cries that struck me then as all the more twisted since it was my family's search for "help" that led me to bring her there in the first place. I know that tying Todd to a bed won't help his illness and will, in fact, make him more resistant to seeking treatment going forward. Merle's encounters with forced treatment traumatized her and only increased her resolve to avoid seeing doctors.

• • •

After the Code Green team straps Todd down, and after the security and medical teams debrief about the use of restraints (standard policy whenever force is used), Dr. McGhee pulls on blue examination gloves and enters the seclusion room. "I would really like to know if you have any injuries," she says.

"*You* did this to me," Todd fumes through his spit mask. "You're going to pay for it."

"Okay," she replies, nodding, although he can't see her.

After an hour, during which Todd has been closely watched in the seclusion room, the pills have left him sedated, and Dr. McGhee proceeds with the exam. "I'm going to listen to your heart," she says. He doesn't respond.

Many experts adamantly oppose restraints as a barbaric relic of earlier times. "In England, they've largely not used restraints for over two hundred years," explains Elyn Saks, a USC law professor with chronic schizophrenia whose story we'll hear more about later. "We should be able to do the same things." Others see restraints as a necessary evil—the only way to ensure patient and staff safety in a dangerous situation—especially in today's EDs when patients may be intoxicated, they may carry weapons, or their psychosis may make them combative. Forty-seven percent of emergency physicians report having been physically assaulted while at work.[1] When a patient like Todd is physically acting out against staff, what choice do they have?

LAC+USC psych ED director Dr. Dias sees today's use of restraints as characteristically different from that of years past. "Four hundred years ago, people would stay chained up for a lifetime. Nowadays, they stay 'chained up' for four hours or less, and in that four-hour window we give them medication that's meant to calm them down and get them to a state of mind where we can actually release them." Even so, you couldn't ask for a more potent symbol of our failure to communicate, connect, and seek collaborative care.

• • •

How did Todd, Johanna, Monte, and Merle get ill? In general, why do people develop mental illness? Whether it's genes, environment, upbringing, or disease, the question has intrigued and perplexed scientists and philosophers alike. The truth is, we don't know, but it's increasingly apparent that there's an interplay of influences in every case, not just a single trigger.

1. Nature and Nurture

Recent science has made clear that biological factors play a major role in the development of SMI. Since the 1970s, we have known that a considerable risk is inherited.[2] Since the 1960s, experts found that certain gene variants—as opposed to home environment—heighten the risk by comparing the outcomes of: identical twins who were adopted by parents without psychotic disorders, fraternal twins raised apart, and children adopted into a family where one parent had schizophrenia. Identical twins of people with schizophrenia have about a 50 percent chance of developing the disease, and nonidentical (or dizygotic) twins have a 20 percent chance of both having the disease.[3] Although environmental factors can play a role, individuals don't *learn* to develop a disease such as schizophrenia. That is, being raised by a nonbiological parent with schizophrenia does not increase someone's risk of the disease. New studies affirm the role of biology.[4]

Twenty-first-century advances in genetics such as the Human Genome Project have also shown that genetic risk may account for a substantial likelihood of developing SMI. When we talk about genetic risk, it's important to understand that you don't have to inherit a certain gene or piece of DNA; the risk can come from epigenetic mutations in the womb or after birth. More than a hundred areas on the human genome may increase the risk for schizophrenia, and just as many may be responsible for mood disorders such as bipolar disorder and depression.

A large study published in 2018 in the journal *Science* vividly illustrates the complex biological realities of psychiatric diseases.[5] The authors' review of DNA from more than one million people found that similar risk factors can be found in the presence of *many* serious psychiatric diseases. In other words, they may not be distinct disease states at all; instead, clinical presentations or symptoms can result from similar genetic vulnerabilities.

As geneticist Ben Neale, PhD, at the Broad Institute of MIT and Harvard explains, "The same common genetic risk landscape is in part shared with basically every other major form of psychopathology [using the current DSM classifications]." This is in contrast to neurological diagnoses like Parkinson's or Huntington's disease, each of which has distinct chromosomal abnormalities. Does this speak to our imprecise and insufficient diagnostic categories? Will psychiatric diseases eventually be classified by their genetic alterations and not their symptoms? If such defining biological and genetics discoveries are made, will these diseases cease to be considered psychiatric and instead be called neurological conditions? Or are most psychiatric diseases mainly due to the complex interplay between our psychology and that abstract entity we call *the mind*, such that SMI will never be traced to distinct biological or physical etiologies, unlike neurological or other brain diseases?

From my own experience, I believe that the most disordered states of mind have a biological basis, meaning that some people are born with or develop, through unknown mechanisms, malfunctioning biological systems in their brains. For some people, the biological malformation may be so strong that disease cannot be avoided. But for most of those vulnerable people, developing destructive diseases is ultimately due to a complex interaction of their biology, experiences, psychology, and culture.

In addition to genetics, inflammation may play a significant role. Inflammation refers to the body's response to perceived invaders such as bacteria, viruses, or parasites, or, in the case of autoimmune diseases, when the perceived invader is a normal part of the person's body. In the early twentieth century, scientists found that some cases of insanity resulted from advanced syphilis, a sexually transmitted bacterial infection caused by the spirochete *Treponema pallidum*. Thirty percent of those who go untreated for more than a decade progress into tertiary syphilis.[6] In this severe form of the disease, the infection can infiltrate and damage the brain and nerves in what is called neurosyphilis, leading to symptoms of schizophrenia-like delusions, depression with suicidal intent, personality change and aggressiveness, and dementia-like memory loss. Inspired by the discovery of syphilis-caused insanity—and its eventual cure by penicillin—twentieth-century doctors optimistically looked for other infectious causes of SMI, although no others seemed to have such an undeniable cause and effect, and that thread of research was largely dropped by the mid-1900s.

For the past decade, Dr. Torrey has argued that, on the contrary, we have overlooked several biological influences on SMI. *Toxoplasma gondii*, a parasite that lives in cats and other felines and can cause the toxoplasmosis infection, affects the dopamine-containing brain cells that are strongly implicated in psychosis. The theory is supported by epidemiological data that shows that adults with psychosis had more contact with cats as children.[7] Evidence also suggests that probiotics can repair the bacterial equilibrium in the gut, modulate immune function, and improve symptoms in individuals with schizophrenia.[8]

One of the most significant breakthroughs in understanding possible biological mechanisms in schizophrenia came in 2016, when Harvard researchers Beth Stevens, PhD, and Steven McCarroll, PhD, determined that certain genes implicated in immune system response seem to be altered in some people with schizophrenia.[9] Not only that, they found evidence that an overactive immune response may chip off brain connections in the frontal lobes, aggressively deleting brain cells beyond what typically occurs during the normal process of late-adolescent brain maturation called *pruning*. (More on this later.)

Although genes, inflammation, infection, and even brain injuries incurred during childbirth or head injuries accumulated on the sports field are all increasingly likely SMI factors,[10] developing a psychiatric disease seems to require more than biology; many experts believe there is some sort of trigger for the seed of mental illness to take root. It could be childhood trauma, abnormally high levels of stress, substance abuse, or poverty. And, of course, these things compound. Depression, psychosis, stress, and anxiety disrupt the biological mechanisms of the brain's emotional, reasoning, and cognitive centers, and the longer they go untreated, the worse their impact. Stress also damages the key structures of the brain and decreases the size of the memory center called the hippocampus.[11] The vicious cycle of untreated psychiatric disorders causes more brain dysfunction, which leads to poor decision making, damaged relationships, diminished circumstances, and, you guessed it, more depression, confusion, chaos, and stress.

2. Poverty and Trauma

Poverty, jail, substance abuse, and stress can cause a budding mental illness to develop into its most lethal forms. "Poor people with serious illnesses who don't have support are very likely to end up either in jails, or rotating in and out of hospitals and homelessness," researcher and psychiatry professor Jeanne Miranda, PhD, tells me. "The more that patients have social factors impeding their ability to function in the world, the worse their outcomes are going to be, no matter what treatments we give them." Such factors include access to housing, meaningful work or other activities, community and connection with others, medical care, and nutritious food. "All of those things are essential to form a true treatment for someone, and it's completely ignored in our system, for the most part," Dr. Miranda says. In her experience, one of the most effective ways to improve the lives of people with SMI is to ensure that one single person in the mental health system sticks by them for the long haul, rather than bouncing them between offices and agencies and caregivers. That is true of all ailments, but perhaps more so with SMI than with an illness like heart disease in which there are curative steps, such as arterial bypass surgery, that can help even in advanced stages of the disease. An illness such as schizophrenia has no such end-stage cure.

Mental illness can lead to poverty, but does poverty cause mental illness? Nothing is straightforward when it comes to SMI, but Jeffrey Draine, PhD, and his coauthors of the paper "Role of Social Disadvantage in Crime, Joblessness, and Homelessness among Persons with Serious Mental Illness" explain the common downward spiral this way: "If persons with mental illness are not poor to begin with they are likely to become poor, and poverty factors become salient in explaining common outcomes such as quality of life, social and occupational functioning, general health, and psychiatric symptoms." The bottom line is that socioeconomic stress is correlated with and contributes to the development of many categories of mental illness.[12]

3. Substance Abuse

Mental illness and substance abuse feed each other
until you have a conflagration that is much more toxic
than the sum of its parts. If having a mental illness is like
living in a house with a smoldering fire in the basement,
substance abuse is like hurling in live grenades from the
second floor. It makes everything exponentially worse.

Dr. Dixon pioneered findings in the area of what are
now referred to as *co-occurring diagnoses* (meaning SMI
combined with a substance use disorder [SUD]). She
began studying this when we were both residents in 1989,
confirming "the alarmingly high rate of substance abuse"
among people with schizophrenia.[13] Since then,
significant research has called into question the false
binary between SMI and SUD. At least one quarter of
people struggling with homelessness also have an SMI,[14]
and within that subset, as many as two thirds also have a
primary substance use disorder or other chronic health
condition.

Co-occurring SUDs are also found in about one
quarter of all individuals with SMI,[15] and the catalytic
factor isn't always hard drugs bought on seedy street
corners. I once treated a brilliant student from an affluent
family attending an Ivy League college who, after
spending her junior semester abroad in Amsterdam
smoking as much weed as she could, developed the
symptoms of schizophrenia. Her intense exposure to
marijuana had opened a window on psychosis that I
couldn't close. She was no longer able to handle the most
basic college courses and had to drop out of school. She
became paranoid, her thoughts disorganized, and she felt
increasingly isolated from friends. Ultimately, after a

decade of medication and therapy, her condition improved, and she was able to return to college to earn her degree. Medicine, psychotherapy, and avoidance of all substances of abuse enabled her to restore her sanity. She was extremely fortunate to have had well-heeled parents with plenty of resources to draw upon to help her recover; many don't.

• • •

A year after the ED fiasco, Todd is back in skid row, the neighborhood that he's called home since he arrived here from Illinois in 1989. Todd has rejoined the 53,195 homeless people in Los Angeles County and 31,516 in the city of Los Angeles,[16] at least 27 percent of whom are believed to have an SMI.

Talking over wailing police sirens and the rumble of a jackhammer gnawing away at the pavement, Todd plays tour guide, pointing out shelters, free clinics, and other social service facilities. On San Pedro Street, people congregate outside the Union Rescue Mission, which helps "men, women, and children escape the streets of skid row through food, shelter, education, counseling, and long-term recovery programs," its façade built of cement blocks painted aqua. A man perches atop a large duffel bag, elbows on his knees. A slender young woman in a ponytail and a gray hoodie sits on a milk crate beside a shopping cart, a "tall boy" beer can on the sidewalk at her feet. Men in wheelchairs loiter outside a long chain of tents pitched on the sidewalk. A woman sells used clothing laid out in piles on a tarp. A twenty-something woman with bleached blond hair in jeans and a spaghetti-strap tank top tosses something small, it's unclear what, into the air, then traipses away, her bare feet blackened with dirt. Above the row of shopping carts, suitcases, and other baggage covered with blankets and tarps hovers a red heart-shaped balloon on a string. Todd occasionally waves hi or asks people how they are doing today.

Todd mentions a woman he knows—"a little sweetheart" who "has a lot of mental health issues." Although a social service organization helped her find housing, she couldn't stay. "She hated living inside so much that she gave it up to be homeless," he explains. "There are documentaries regarding that issue—about people who've been homeless for so many years they prefer to be homeless. Someone like that has got to have mental health issues—when you can't live indoors for whatever reason."

In the decade and a half that Todd has spent on skid row, he's become an expert on the available services: where to get a free shower, wash clothing for $1.25, see a doctor, take an art or life-skills coping class, get counseling, or exchange one dirty needle for five clean ones. That last service might have helped him had he availed himself of it earlier in life: "I caught HIV from shooting drugs," he says. "I was shooting drugs behind somebody that had it and never told me, and I ended up catching it." He explains this with resignation, just a tinge of bitterness showing in the way he sets his jaw. Todd was diagnosed in 2005 when he was hospitalized for pneumonia. "Who gets pneumonia in July? In California, eighty, ninety, one hundred degrees? Pneumonia's one of the biggest killers for people with HIV and AIDS," Todd says. "So, that's why I always wear coats. It could be seventy, eighty degrees out, I got a coat on, you know, 'cause I'm afraid of catching pneumonia."

Now, Todd is prescribed a daily cocktail of HIV medications as well as antipsychotics and mood stabilizers. For a while, he says, doctors were "guinea-pigging me," trying out different combinations of drugs. But over time they found "a nice mellow pattern, I guess, of psychiatric medications to keep me calm. I mean, sure, they keep me calm to a certain extent. They stop the thoughts." His thoughts "jump around" a lot so that he "can't remember short things. I mean, my short-term memory is shot. I could take my medication, and then twenty minutes from now I'll forget that I took my medication, and I'll take more medication. You know what I mean? That's why it's good to have somebody—anybody—to go, 'Wait a minute. You just took your medication, dummy.'"

Monthly visits with a psychiatrist at the outpatient clinic of the LAC+USC Medical Center help keep Todd on track, somewhat. At the very least, the appointments allow him to vent. "Well, how are you doing?" the psychiatrist begins, on a visit that I attend. The date is February 1.

"Today's a fucked-up day," Todd replies. "Today's the anniversary of Maria's death. Remember my girlfriend?"

"Yes."

"The one they tried"—Todd stumbles over his words—"they tried charging me with her murder?"

"Yes. They have a lot to learn. That's ridiculous," says the psychiatrist. "I'm sorry. I really am."

Together, the two of them do the math and realize it's been four years since Maria overdosed while she and Todd were living together in a single room occupancy (SRO) hotel nearby. "You're right. Four years. Oh, my God. Time flies when you're having fun, huh?"

Todd tells his psychiatrist the latest news in his seemingly endless quest to secure a decent apartment. For several months, he has been working with LAMP (now called the People Concern), a nonprofit that helps people who are homeless. He hopes that housing support will afford him the opportunity to save a little money, so he can get his life back on track. "Subsidized housing is great. Everybody thinks we want a free ride. No, we don't want a free ride. We just want a step up. You know what I mean?"

But the stress of this protracted process is particularly overwhelming for Todd. "They keep telling me one thing and another. I feel like a Ping-Pong ball. It's so damned fuckin' hard, and I get pissed off," he says. The leather jacket he's wearing, despite the warm office, squeaks as he shifts in his chair. "It depresses me. And, you know, a lot of shit goes in my head when I get depressed, and the next thing you know"—he interrupts himself with a chuckle and raises his eyebrows—"the sheriffs are being called." His smile reveals a mix of humor and resignation. "This whole trying-to-do-things-normal is frustrating the hell out of me. Because I'm not normal. The government, the system, everybody wants to keep you down. If you're poor, if you're crazy, they want to keep you down, or lock you up. I mean, how many years have I been with Mental Health? Forty-three years and they still haven't fixed me."

Todd has been struggling to eat on the $60 that's left of his $960 monthly disability check after he pays his rent at the SRO where he's managed to find a room this month. Food banks keep him going, but despite his clear intelligence, even organizing the simple tasks necessary to feed himself become a challenge. "I love cereal, so I eat cereal all day long," he tells his psychiatrist. "I have an itty-bitty refrigerator, so I only can buy these milks like this," he says, showing her with his hands. "They're $2, and I only like Ralphs milk, so I have to go all the way to Ralphs to get it. And I gotta get, like, one of those every day. It costs $2.19. I go get one, even if I have to, like, go borrow a couple dollars or something, I get one of those 'cause I love cereal." Then, like a little kid proud of mastering some new stunt, he tells her excitedly about how this morning he used a trick he'd learned in prison: substituting yogurt for milk in his cereal. "I got a thing of yogurt from the food bank. I bought a cantaloupe. So I had cantaloupe slices I put in the yogurt, and orange I put in the yogurt, and . . ." He racks his brain to remember. "Banana! I put it in the yogurt. I got a big ol' bowl of Cap'n Crunch." He laughs. "And I put the yogurt with all that fruit instead of milk."

"Oh, good!" says his doctor, encouragingly.

"Oh, man, that was good," Todd agrees, smiling.

"That's very creative."

Then, in a flash, he leans over, hand over his eyes, and circles back to Maria. "I was thinking maybe later, I don't know . . . I'm not getting drunk today. I got a couple of bucks. I could go buy a beer and go pour it in our favorite spot." He sits with the idea, deep creases across his forehead. "Because I don't know where she's buried."

"Oh, that's hard."

"I heard they burned her body. You know, she didn't have any relatives." He pauses, eyes wet. "I loved that girl." He nods, lips pursed, eyes far away.

"You did," says his psychiatrist. "I remember your coming together."

"We'd come together like shadows."

After his appointment, Todd stands on the sidewalk in a low-rent business district on the outskirts of skid row. He explains that he no longer has a girlfriend. "I have this fear in my head that being with somebody is . . . you know, I'm jeopardizing their life." But his "friends out on the streets" mean a lot to him. His buddy Ron, for

example, a veteran whom Todd describes lovingly as "a nerd—
legitimately a nerd. All he likes doing is reading. That's all he does
is read, read, read, read." Since Ron lost his library card, he and
Todd alternate days using Todd's. "Today's his day." Friendships
like these help keep him connected and, in some ways, he is much
better off than his neighbors. "When it becomes okay in your mind
to sleep on the ground next to dried-up urine or dried-up feces—
human waste . . . when that's okay—you know you've snapped.
You've gone too far over the cusp of reality. I was there once," he
concedes. "It was prison that pulled me back out of it."

Todd was in his twenties the first time he went to prison. (He
never told me why he was incarcerated and always changed the
subject whenever I brought it up.) Spending two decades "in an
eight-by-twelve cell" is part of why he now prefers to be outside. "I
really don't mind living on the streets, except for having to find a
shower or something—usually a bathroom. 'Cause I used to live on
the streets and dig through garbage cans and all that stuff, and I
was happy." But his HIV status, high viral load, and low T-cell
count leave him susceptible to infection. "Because of my medical
issues, I need to live indoors."

Standing on a street corner across from a row of discount stores
selling caps, dishes, luggage, and liquor store supplies, Todd explains the interminable cycle. "I go back and forth between fighting and running, fighting and running, fighting and running.
Right now, I'm fighting again, probably because of my medical
situation. I don't want to die on the streets." He pauses, then shrugs.
"A lot of people out here suffer from either drug addiction or mental health issues and that's why they're down here." His voice cracks.
"It's sad—it's really sad," he says, the tears and anger welling up.
"And I suffer from it, and these people suffer from it, and there ain't

no help nowhere! We just keep going around in circles, and we get nothing. It's just sad."

Three months later, Todd's stress boils over after a phone call with his LAMP housing counselor, Steve Mitchell, who has been working for months on his behalf. Todd is still waiting for safe, affordable housing to come through. Finally, Mitchell tells him that LAMP has not only received the necessary payment voucher but also found an available unit—but Todd can't move in for a few more days. "It makes no sense to me, man," Todd says as he hangs up the phone. "Leave someone sleeping on the goddamned sidewalk when he's got a fucking apartment."

With a high-pitched wail, he hurls his precious phone onto the pavement, pieces of it flying. "I've heard the same thing three fucking times," he moans, pacing, arms flailing. "Roof! Fucking homeless on the fucking sidewalk when he's got a goddamned, a fucking roof." His words come out choked and garbled. "He's got a fucking roof. And he can't get in it. He fucking can't get in it." Todd folds at the waist, doubled over, fists pounding at the air. His sunglasses drop to the ground. "I don't understand it," he yells, struggling to pick up his belongings and shove them into his pockets. "I don't fucking understand it. Motherfuckers!"

The next day, Mitchell comes through, and Todd turns a key in the door to his new apartment—a clean, well-kept studio, complete with a couch, a bed, a kitchenette, and a private bathroom tiled in bright teal. "It's nice," says Mitchell as the door swings open.

"It's a big one! Yay!" Todd says, wearing a huge smile. He laughs as he walks over to the wide picture window overlooking the street, then begins to rock slightly, back and forth.

"Congratulations," says Mitchell, smiling.

When Todd turns around it's clear that he's weeping. He sits down on the window ledge. "Four years, man," he says, crying, shaking his head, smiling at Mitchell. "Four years." He wipes his eyes, but tears keep coming. "Thank you, Steve. Thank you."

Two years later, I find Todd's name on a roster of Los Angeles County jail arrests. He appears at his court hearing in navy blue scrubs printed with white letters: LA COUNTY JAIL. Limping, wearing a neck brace, and using a walker, he makes his way to the chair beside the public defender, who asks the judge for Todd to be released on his own recognizance "on compassionate grounds" because of his declining T-cell count and the fact that his offense (a small hand-to-hand drug sale) was nonviolent. Because of Todd's previous conviction, the judge denies the request. It takes three months for Todd to accumulate enough in disability checks to post the $1,000 bail necessary to secure his release.

Then Todd loses the apartment, the best home he's had in decades. As Mitchell explains it to me, Todd had put down a deposit on a new place, but it never materialized. Instead the money disappeared. "A scam," says Mitchell. In the meantime, Todd told the building management he was leaving, so they gave his place to someone else. Like most things with Todd, the story doesn't make complete sense. For me, it's confusing; for Todd, the world must seem completely illogical. The last time I saw Todd was outside a Starbucks near skid row, near his run-down SRO. The LA sun was hot, yet Todd wore a heavy corduroy jacket and drank hot coffee to stay warm. Hunched over, thin and weak and fifty-five (the age Merle died), he said he has liver and kidney cancer and is skin-popping heroin for the pain. He smiles, thanks me for the coffee, and gives no sign that he's given up.

CHAPTER 5

"MY SON DIED WITH HIS CIVIL LIBERTIES INTACT"

After observing the sometimes useless, often tragic, intrusion of law enforcement into the lives of people like Monte and Todd, I began to wonder if the law could in fact be used to *help* them instead. In Los Angeles, and across America, we warehouse people with mental illness in jails after court hearings that may last only a few minutes. But there is also a tradition—and now a renewed movement—of using the courts as a path for treatment.

"When you're carrying a hammer, everything looks like a nail, and when you're a judge carrying a gavel, everyone looks like a defendant," says Judge Oscar Kazen, his deep voice hinting at his Texas roots. Today, he says he enjoys doing more than just banging his gavel to consign the convicted to punishment. "We get to help people." Modeling their efforts after the drug courts that compel substance abuse treatment rather than incarceration, he and colleagues established a court to help people follow prescribed treatment.[1]

Early in his career as an attorney, Kazen thought, "You have the right, if you want, to stand on the corner all day long and stare at the sun. As long as you're not hurting anybody, you can go right ahead and do it." But once he got onto the bench, he came to see personal-autonomy rhetoric as, at least in part, a societal cop-out. "It's a much easier thing to wrap your arms around civil liberties and not have to spend the money on treatment courts and placing people in long-term or at least significant treatment for seriously mentally ill individuals so that they can somehow make wellness their habit instead of illness." Although he's "not advocating restraint on liberty for anybody that's seriously mentally ill," he insists that human decency ultimately requires "some more rigorous form of treatment rather than the revolving door that we now have."

Kazen is one of a half dozen judges I've spoken with who are employing what is referred to as *therapeutic jurisprudence.* From New York to Miami to Los Angeles, judges are revisiting the ethics of mandated treatment, which had fallen out of favor since the 1960s. For those individuals with SMI who've committed a crime, there are mental health courts (MHCs) whereby the judge diverts someone convicted of a misdemeanor or felony toward comprehensive treatment instead of jail. (More on MHCs in the next chapter.) Then there's assisted outpatient treatment (AOT), designed to help people who don't have criminal charges pending but have demonstrated difficulty engaging with treatment and avoiding the hospital (and often have extensive arrest histories as well). AOT is for people who are not facing jail but desperately require, yet struggle to adhere to, treatment.

AOT is a less drastic option for leveraging treatment than conservatorships or guardianships. A conservator or guardian is authorized by law to make medical and financial decisions on behalf of an adult who can't maintain his or her own health and safety. For adults with SMI who pose a grave danger to themselves and/or others, a conservator assumes, for varying lengths of time, the kinds of decision-making power that parents have over minors. The conservator is usually a local relative or a trained professional from a registry held by the state. Conservatorships are often initiated by family members at their wits' end or by a medical team at a psychiatric hospital that deems a patient in urgent need of extended treatment that the patient would otherwise resist. The arrangement resembles a hostile takeover of someone's autonomy, and the whole matter is often fraught with suspicions and conflicts. The conservatorship requires continual court appearances, lawyer meetings, substantial fees, and never-ending paperwork.

Although I had long known about these drastic measures to force treatment, I never felt they were an option for my sister. While my mother was alive, it certainly would not have been possible. After her passing, when Merle was living alone, I considered the possibility. Perhaps I could have had the police take Merle to the hospital and then applied for a conservatorship. But arguing my case would not have been easy. Still, looking back—and like almost every family member I know who's lost a loved one tells me—I wish I had tried.

New York's AOT program was established by Kendra's Law, named after a woman who was fatally shoved into the path of a moving subway train by a man with paranoid schizophrenia who had previously refused treatment. Under the law, New York State judges have mandated treatment, including medication, for more than 25,000 people since its implementation in 1999.[2] As Carolyn D. Gorman, previously the project manager for mental illness policy and education policy at the Manhattan Institute, wrote in the *New York Post*, "Leaving those who are seriously mentally ill—who are vulnerable and often homeless, victims of violence themselves or institutionalized in jails and prisons—without treatment is an ethical failure, as well as a safety issue."[3]

In Summit County, Ohio, probate judge Elinore Marsh Stormer ran a mental health court (MHC) in 2000, geared toward helping people with psychiatric disorders who had committed a crime. Judge Stormer tells me, "We were missing the civil piece where people didn't have to get arrested to get mental health treatment." The program, called New Day Court, serves people who have been civilly committed to a psychiatric hospital. Following their hospital discharge, Judge Stormer assigns each individual a case manager from a community treatment center who helps provide the resources necessary for recovery. "Do you need housing? Do you need clothes? Do you need food? Do you need to see a medical doctor as well as a psychiatrist?" The case manager's job is to help provide it, enabling individuals to get back on their feet. Meanwhile, as opposed to the business-as-usual approach whereby courts, hospitals, judges, and doctors wash their hands of the patient and their family after someone with SMI is deemed competent to rejoin society, Judge Stormer examines the treatment plans to make sure they have a reasonable chance of success, and follows up with periodic conferences to confirm that participants are engaged with the process.

Unlike in a mental health court for people with untreated psychiatric disorders and a Drug Court for people with untreated addictions where a judge can incarcerate a noncompliant participant for committing a crime, an AOT court order cannot be the basis for putting someone in jail if they refuse medical care. So, the person with SMI won't face jail time for noncompliance but can be forced into inpatient care. "All I can do is threaten people with hospitalization," Judge Stormer says, but since "nobody wants to be in the hospital," that is often incentive enough. She takes advantage of "what we lovingly call the *black robe effect*": the power of the bench to influence behavior.

In Texas, Judge Kazen also puts the black robe effect to good use. Many people confronting the choice between AOT or continued hospitalization will agree to AOT, he tells me. During his decade presiding over Bexar County's AOT, he has seen the life-changing power and positive impact of leveraged treatment. "Surprisingly, for most of the people who go through that assisted outpatient treatment, that small crack of a door opens. Because after about six months on the order, you develop a relationship with them. They realize, 'Wow. These people are really here to help me. They're really not trying to throw me in jail.' It's kind of like what happened with Eric."

Eric Smith had been diagnosed with bipolar disorder as a teenager. Before the diagnosis, Eric explains, he'd "had no way of knowing that how I felt was out of the norm in any way." The news of his disease left him both disappointed and relieved that there was a name for what he was going through. As Eric's illness progressed throughout his twenties, he was prescribed basically every drug psychiatry had to offer, including mood stabilizers, benzodiazepines, and antidepressants. Sometimes he felt the medications helped but other times not. Bothered by side effects and generally unconvinced, Eric occasionally skipped doses or stopped taking his prescriptions entirely. At times, he lost faith in the idea that any treatment could help. "I have been on everything under the sun and every time a new med comes out, I'm on that and here I am, still bipolar and in a bad state," he recalls thinking at the time.

For years, Eric self-medicated with street drugs ("the only thing that I never, ever touched was heroin"), which led to a co-occurring SUD. "I know that might sound like a cop-out for someone to do drugs but I'm telling you, my mind was chaos unless I was using. Not that it wasn't chaos when I was using, but it certainly made me *feel* like it wasn't chaos," he tells me. The drugs gave him "a peace of mind that none of the meds I had been prescribed" managed to offer. He wound up in rehab in 2006, at age twenty-three.

Two years later, he was sober, but his mind was cycling between depressive lows and manic highs, despite taking his prescribed medications. Before he wound up in jail, he had been awake for nearly three days. "My body was tired; my mind was tired but simultaneously the 'up' side of me was winning and I couldn't sleep." His head was a swirl of grandiosity, impulsivity, racing thoughts, and delusions. "I believed that I was working along with the FBI. I believed I was part of the CIA. I believed I was part of the Secret Service."

In addition, despite not being in a romantic relationship, Eric was "under the impression that I needed to find a bride immediately. 'If I need a bride, I need diamond rings,'" he thought. He walked into a jewelry store and bought an engagement ring and a wedding band. (Excessive and impulsive spending often occur during the manic phase of bipolar disease.)

"Then I went to go show my parents that I got these diamonds." For weeks, Eric's parents had been growing increasingly more worried, with no idea how to help or keep him safe. When they finally reached a psychiatrist who had worked with their son previously, the doctor urged them to admit their son to a psychiatric facility. The best way to do this would be to have him arrested, the idea being that the police would quickly transfer him from jail to a mental hospital for observation. Unlike Monte's family, Eric's parents may have been less worried about involving law enforcement given that their son was white. Still, things did not go as planned.

For several days prior to his jewelry spree, Eric had become increasingly hostile toward his parents. He began making threats and, in accordance with the psychiatrist's advice, they issued a restraining order against him, knowing that if he violated the order, he would be arrested. He challenged his father to "go ahead and call the police," Eric says, "and then I went and sat down on their porch until the police showed up and arrested me. I made no attempts to resist arrest."

What happened next was "horrendous." At the police station, he was stripped of his clothes and left naked in a cell "in the midst of a bipolar delusional meltdown." Officers ordered him to spread his buttocks and lift his scrotum so they could look for contraband. "It was a dehumanizing experience from the very beginning." To this day, Eric identifies deeply with people who are incarcerated, no matter if they've broken the law or if mental illness isn't a factor. "It was horrible."

Things grew worse when he was transferred to the San Antonio jail, where officers in riot gear and helmets would run into the holding pens to break up the near-constant fights. The jail did not carry his prescribed psychiatric medications, so he remained inadequately treated for the month he spent behind bars. His agitation worsened to the point that the authorities transferred him from a room of thirty people to a solitary cell where he remained isolated for twenty-three hours a day. On two separate occasions, he recalled being allowed in a common area for fifteen minutes. "After that, police and inmates told me I was making people nervous, so they kept me isolated in that solitary cell thereafter. There was a window and I could occasionally hear TV or people talking," Eric tells me. Otherwise, "I was by myself just decompensating in a jail cell."

His decline left him in such bad shape that guards at one point refused to let his parents see him although they'd waited hours for the chance. Corrections officers told them that he was potentially dangerous. "I'm told that led to my mom crying pretty bad," Eric says. "She wanted to see me, and she knew I was in a bad place. Luckily, there was an officer there who had a family member who also had a serious mental illness. He understood the scenario and I guess he pulled rank. My parents were finally able to come see me. Everything in jail, everything, other than the occasional compassionate, understanding officer, it was a just a nightmare."

Eric's incarceration did ultimately lead to treatment, however. Jail officials had been telling his parents that no hospital bed was available and that they were preparing to release him onto the streets. But at the eleventh hour, after a tremendous effort by his family and a social worker at the jail, he was admitted to a psychiatric hospital. He was the most ill he'd ever been. Convinced he worked for the Secret Service, Smith heard the voice of then CIA director General David Petraeus issuing orders.

Over the course of Eric's three-month hospital stay, his medications were adjusted, his condition was stabilized, and his symptoms finally receded. He was transferred, under the Bexar County AOT program, there called Involuntary Outpatient Care (IOPC), to a group home that "had lots of rules," including mandated medication.

Seven years after graduating from his AOT court order in San Antonio, Eric, now thirty-six, tells me that court-ordered treatment revolutionized the management of his disease. He attributes his turnaround to the consistent and comprehensive care provided by a team of doctors, nurses, public defenders, case workers, licensed counselors, and the judge—an approach that's called *wraparound care.* The specialist teams check in with each other every week in an effort to make sure that providers are coordinating their care, keeping their clients engaged in treatment, and helping clients reintegrate into the community. As in any therapeutic relationship, chemistry is everything. Smith accepted the intervention by Judge Kazen in part because of his warm and caring attitude. Judge Kazen makes no bones about the intensity of the program for participants. "We're going to get into this person's life," he says. Even so, most cooperate.

Lawyer Brian Stettin, policy director at the Treatment Advocacy Center who crafted AOT law for twenty years, takes it a step further and says most people "enter the program happily and are not refusing treatment at the time the order is imposed. Typically, they are coming directly from a hospital stay, are reasonably stable, and see AOT as their ticket out of the hospital."

Since the Bexar County program's inception, Judge Kazen says that participants have spent more than two thirds fewer days in hospitals than their counterparts who aren't enrolled. Eric has not been hospitalized since he graduated from AOT in 2012. He says that AOT "not only saved my life but changed the entire trajectory of what my life was like." He has since transformed from someone who "wasn't a participant in reality," into a graduate student pursuing a master of social work degree, with the goal of becoming a licensed clinical social worker (LCSW). Far from an infringement on his civil liberties, Eric credits AOT for his own recovery and has since become a public spokesperson for leveraged treatment.

Today, forty-seven states and the District of Columbia authorize some form of AOT.[4] Leveraged treatment reduces hospitalization, arrest and incarceration, homelessness, and violent acts associated with mental illness, as well as increasing treatment adherence and easing caregiver stress and strain.[5] In addition to quality-of-life improvements, it also significantly reduces costs associated with the cycling of people with SMI through emergency rooms, psychiatric hospitals, and jails.[6]

Advocates say the programs save lives, reducing crimes both by and against people with psychiatric illnesses, as well as suicides. Critics say they return us to a day when psychiatrists arbitrarily decided who is normal and who isn't, when diagnoses enforced by a decree from a judge or the state could land a person in an institution for life just for being different. Whichever side you're on, it's important to acknowledge that in AOT, the word *assisted* is a euphemism. Although the specifics vary by state, when the treatment is ordered by a judge, it never feels totally voluntary.

If you're like me, alarm bells go off when you hear that a judge, even with the guidance of a mental health professional, can define the limits of mental health and force someone to take psychiatric medications. As a teenager, I was drawn to the eloquence of those who championed personal freedom over some culturally sanctioned definition of normalcy: Michel Foucault, R. D. Laing, and a personal favorite of mine, American psychiatrist Thomas Szasz, MD. In his landmark 1961 article for *American Psychologist* and his subsequent book, *The Myth of Mental Illness: Foundations of a Theory of Personal Conduct*, Dr. Szasz argued that the term *mental illness* refers to "undesirable thoughts, feelings and behaviors" rather than "a demonstrable biological process that affects the bodies of living organisms."

So impressed by him, I wrote to Dr. Szasz at age eighteen, hoping for a job. But in 1975, he had no use for an undergrad seeking a summer internship. Instead, summer after my freshman year of college, I did research at Friends Hospital, America's first private psychiatric hospital (and Merle's third hospital), which was about two miles from my home. There I studied people with SMI who didn't accept that they had an illness. (Although this was a hospital where, two years earlier, I had dropped Merle off for electroshock treatment, I kept the family secret, never telling anyone I worked with about my sister.)

One night, after a long day at the hospital, I attended the lecture of another humanist psychologist speaking to a packed house in Philly's Rittenhouse Square. He'd written a number of brilliant books about psychotherapy that I'd read, reread, and revered. I loved what he said about how we could free ourselves from the scripts we live by despite how they constrain us and not be needlessly constricted, pathologized, diagnosed, and pigeonholed by the psychiatric establishment. Sitting there, I wondered how humanistic psychology might apply to my sister, who that year had jumped out the window and was now recuperating in my parents' bed. At the end of his talk, in this groovy room of downtown intellectuals, I decided to raise my hand and ask a question. I dared not mention my sister but asked the esteemed author more generally about how his theories about psychotherapy might apply to people with psychosis. He responded that he'd *never seen a psychotic.* He believed psychosis was just a label imposed by psychiatrists who wanted to control and categorize their patients. *Psychosis didn't exist* was a Szaszian view with which I was well acquainted. *Had he never ventured onto a psych ward? Could he fathom what it was like to love someone like Merle, who, by the way, agreed that her diagnosis was a fallacy?* I realized that, ingenious though he may have been, my role model didn't know what the hell he was talking about. The "myth of mental illness" may sound good on paper, may even be fine if you're treating the "worried well" or some neurotic college student like me. It is, of course, a social good to resist the deeply harmful labels imposed by authoritarian doctors over the course of our country's history, whether labeling homosexuality a disease, as the APA did until 1973, or blaming "refrigerator mothers" for their children's autism until the 1960s. But the "myth of mental illness" doesn't wash for the many cases I have seen, nor help people who are suffering.

That said, the debate between coercive treatment and civil liberty is an essential one. What sways me toward the former in many situations is both my personal and my clinical experience. When it comes to their own family members experiencing mental illness and/or substance abuse, many of the most ardent civil rights advocates I know recognize the importance of guardianships, conservatorships, and court-mandated treatment to prevent more harm coming to their loved ones. I watched my sister die after a lifetime of what amounted to neglect in my eyes. There are no easy answers here: How can we respect personal autonomy among people who resist treatment and deny their illness? Where do we draw the line between giving everyone full civil liberties and allowing a psychotic disease to run the show? Is there a logical and proper role for the courts to help those who are being held captive by their own minds?

One person who makes a persuasive argument for therapeutic jurisprudence is Norm Ornstein, a noted political scholar and my colleague in mental health advocacy. His opinions on the matter stem from losing his son. Here is the story that he and his wife, Judy Harris, a Washington lawyer, generously shared with me:

Matthew Ornstein's troubles began in 2005, when he had a psychotic episode at age twenty-four. Before then, he had been a warm, funny, popular, and empathetic young man. In high school, he won national championships in debate, then went on to excel at Princeton. After graduation, he moved to Hollywood with the dream of becoming a writer and stand-up comic, co-creating a television show for the National Lampoon Network that VH1 was considering picking up. Then, all of a sudden (or so it seemed at the time), he became withdrawn and occasionally delusional, alternating between deep depression and euphoria. His emerging illness soon took on a religious quality.

Not long after the onset of his disease, Matthew refused to stay in a hotel room with the number six, a symbol of the devil, on the door and, because no other room was available, wound up sleeping in the car. On another occasion, he drove all the way from Washington, D.C., to the outskirts of Boston, for the wedding of a college friend, but when he noticed that the license plate on the car in front of him contained sixes, he turned around, drove all the way back to Washington, and then set out once more for Massachusetts.

Despite his increasingly bizarre behavior, Matthew did not think he was sick. Instead, he believed that he had done something to anger God, so God had "put him in the penalty box," taking his soul and leaving his body behind while deciding whether to come for Matthew's body next or return his soul. Matthew spent the next ten years trying to redeem himself and earn back God's love through strict religious practices and acts of charity. He rejected out of hand the notion of mental illness, believing that was just a construct meant to constrain behavior that society deemed unacceptable.

After his first psychotic episode, Matthew's life in California deteriorated and he moved back in with his parents on the East Coast. He agreed to see a few doctors in an attempt to allay their concerns,

but despite their ample resources and extensive network of knowledgeable friends and colleagues, his parents were unable to find a
doctor with more than a passing interest in working with Matthew
once he made clear to them that under no circumstances would
he take medicine. He believed that God would deem treatment
with medications as "taking the easy way out," which would impact God's judgment about whether to return his soul.

His family vacillated between pity and protection, tough love
and unconditional love.

After eighteen months of useless doctors' visits, Norm found
Wayne Fenton, MD, a prominent psychiatrist who served as an associate director of NIMH and maintained a part-time private practice. Recognizing that it was senseless to expect seriously ill
individuals to keep weekly appointments in an office, Dr. Fenton
met his patients where they were, both figuratively and literally. In
Matthew's case, that meant at home in bed. For about nine months,
Dr. Fenton would come to their house around nine or ten at night
and Matthew would shout down, "Is he here again? I'm not seeing
him, I'm not seeing anybody." Dr. Fenton would go upstairs anyway and the two would wind up talking for two hours. Their therapeutic relationship seemed to be helping. Judy tells me that
Matthew appeared to be bonding with Dr. Fenton. "He would
come downstairs to dinner after his sessions with the doctor, even
though often it was close to midnight, and he was more talkative
with us on those occasions."

Then, in September 2006, Dr. Fenton was beaten to death at age
fifty-three by a nineteen-year-old with schizophrenia who had
stopped taking his medication. Dr. Fenton had agreed to see that
young man, another doctor's patient, on Labor Day, at a hastily
scheduled visit in an office building that was all but deserted

because of the holiday. (This horrific incident is yet another reason many psychiatrists avoid taking on patients with SMI despite the reality that the patients are far more likely to be the victims of violence than the perpetrators.[7])

Afterward, Matthew saw a few other mental health professionals intermittently (so long as they didn't prescribe medication), but he never again bonded with any practitioner. His mental health continued to decline, and his parents grew more frantic. Early one morning in 2009, the mother of a young woman Matthew had known since elementary school called to tell Judy that Matthew had been obsessively attempting to reach her daughter on her birthday by sending urgent emails and texts throughout the previous night. Judy called the doctor Matthew had been seeing on occasion and asked him to meet her at the family home, where he had been living alone. The doctor working with the family had suggested to his parents that changing Matthew's environment by moving him out of his childhood home might be helpful. Although they had moved to a flat downtown, they had not yet successfully convinced him to join them. But when Matthew opened the door, Judy deeply regretted having let him live alone.

Matthew was thin and disheveled, the house in total disarray, strewn with empty bottles and cans, old pizza boxes, and half-filled food containers. He agreed to let his mother in, on the condition that the doctor leave, and that she join him in the basement. He had a copy of Anne Frank's *The Diary of a Young Girl* and a diary that Judy's mother, who had escaped the Holocaust, had written at around the same age. Matthew told her: "We're going to commemorate the children who died in the Holocaust. Sit with me. We'll read a line from Anne's and then Grandma's diaries," and then he read the names from a list he had, took a puff on a cigarette, and put it out on the carpet.

Judy obliged for a while, and then, saying that she needed to call her office to tell them she wouldn't be coming to work, she went outside, phoned the doctor, asked him to call the police, and then returned. When two police officers arrived, Matthew willingly left with them. After the few days of confinement permitted by law on an emergency basis, the doctors at the hospital applied for a court order enabling them to keep Matthew for treatment, arguing that he was an imminent danger to himself, due to malnourishment and dramatic weight loss from not eating or sleeping.

Before the hearing to commit, Judy was assured by the doctors, much to her great relief, that her testimony wouldn't be needed. Based on that, she promised Matthew that she would not "testify against him." But midway through the hearing, the hospital's counsel appeared in the waiting room and told Judy that "the only hope of keeping Matthew in the hospital for treatment was if I went into the courtroom and testified as to what I had observed on the day I called the police. It was an impossible decision: on the one hand, I knew how badly Matthew needed help but, on the other hand, I had given him my word." Judy convinced herself that if Matthew got treatment but never spoke to her again, she would be able to live with that—so long as he got better. But she will never forget the look in Matthew's eyes when he saw her enter that court-room, the tremor in his voice when he uttered the words: "Mom, you promised." As result of the hearing, Matthew was held at the hospital—but was released just a few weeks later, after appealing to the court, through his lawyer, and successfully blocking the psychiatrists' recommendation for forced medication. Matthew's relationship with his parents never fully recovered.

In the four and a half years that followed, Matthew grew increasingly more paranoid and disconnected from reality as well as isolated, pulling further away from his friends and family, especially his parents, who he felt "never took his side." He traveled the country, but his appearance, heavy smoking, and odd sleeping habits caused his neighbors to avoid him everywhere he moved.

In August 2014, Matthew's parents were able to pinpoint his general location only through his phone, which was still on their family plan. Norm drew up a map of every hotel and motel with smoking rooms within a sixty-mile radius of that dot. They spent Judy's birthday driving from one to the next until they found Matthew's car in the parking lot of the fifty-ninth hotel on their list. They decided not to tell Matthew that they knew where he was, terrified that he would ditch his phone and disappear again. Instead, they tried to reassure themselves that Matthew was in a safe place: a safe hotel, with free breakfast and housekeeping services. Nearly every weekend they made the six-hour round-trip to check on him ("Had his draperies opened? His car been moved?") and they hired a detective to keep a lookout when they could not.

Matthew would still occasionally respond to his parents' texts and messages. But in 2014, he remained silent during the December holidays. By New Year's Day 2015, Norm and Judy had grown increasingly concerned. On January third, they drove for the last time to the motel in Newark, Delaware, that they had been regularly visiting without Matthew's knowledge, arriving at about five o'clock that evening. This time, a squad car was parked outside. Matthew was dead.

During Matthew's junior year of college, which he'd spent at the University of Cape Town in South Africa, he and his roommate would venture out to remote areas to camp. They would sit and talk and marvel at the southern sky. A couple years before his death, Matthew had told his roommate that "whenever I'm feeling anxious or agitated, I set up our old tent and go inside it, and I can sort of feel the peace of those days in South Africa." That peace was likely what Matthew was seeking when he pitched that very tent in his motel room and went inside with a book, his glasses, and a small Coleman lantern. The forensics suggest that he fell asleep, book in hand, glasses and lantern on, and when the lantern ran out of fuel, the propane tank that powered it emitted the carbon monoxide that killed him. A carbon monoxide detector sat on the nightstand, beside it an unopened pack of batteries.

When contemplating the legal provisions that hamstrung their ability to get help—Norm says he viewed his son's "freedom" as a "false freedom—false because [Matthew] was unaware of his own condition and the awful trajectory that it took him on." The "true insanity," as he wrote in the *New York Times* later that year, "is that our laws leave those who suffer to fend for themselves."

Judy puts it even more succinctly: "My son died with his civil liberties intact."

Marvin Swartz, MD, a professor of psychiatry at Duke University and a leader in the study of leveraged treatment's efficacy, tells me that when it comes to civil rights concerns, "people are talking for [other] people." Directly asking people with SMI and their families and clinicians their opinions on mandated care, as Dr. Swartz has done, reveals some unexpected and often unheard perspectives. "Life is full of trade-offs, and this is a trade-off," he says. "Would they be willing to trade off the liberty of not getting treatment if they got the benefits of better housing, safer environment, not being psychotic, not being hospitalized? They say, 'If this is gonna get me out from under a bridge, and I'll have a warm place to live, I don't care about this.' Civil liberties isn't the big thing to people living under bridges."

When evaluating the costs versus benefits of coercive treatment, it's also important to consider the results. In a study of New York State's AOT law, Dr. Swartz says that he found a significant decline in the number of hospitalizations among participants. Part of this is likely due to the obligations of the care institutions within AOT jurisdictions. An important feature of Kendra's Law, for example, is that it makes treatment agencies accountable for patient care. "As much as it commits the patient to treatment, it commits the providers to providing that treatment and not letting the patient get lost," Dr. Swartz says. This entails a serious financial responsibility, but under these programs the judge, treatment team, family, and patient work closely for months or even years to provide the continuity of care that can create a real shift toward overall well-being. Setting aside the moral obligations that we, as a society, have to care for the sick, AOT makes good sense on a cost-savings basis alone. Schwartz's data shows that enrollment decreased hospitalizations, improved medication adherence, decreased violent incidents, and reduced the health costs to taxpayers by 50 percent.

These programs boast encouraging results, but barriers to entry prevent more individuals and their families from benefiting. Awareness is one such roadblock. Although outpatient commitment laws have long been on the books in some states, I—a practicing psychiatrist working for nearly a decade to investigate the lives of people with SMI in this country—had never heard of AOT until recently. Where programs exist, they are designed to have the petitions brought by the treating doctor,[8] hospital, or mental health authority. Although it's rare, in some states, family members can themselves start the AOT process.

I asked Dr. Swartz to walk me through how I, as a family member, might have engaged Merle with AOT, had I been given the chance. "In our state [North Carolina] what you would do is go to the magistrate and swear out your position arguing that your sister is dangerous to herself or unable to care for herself and [therefore] at risk of dying of severe neglect. Once that's issued by the magistrate, the police will pick her up and take her to the emergency room for an examination by a psychiatrist." At that point, "and that's the tricky thing," he says, a psychiatrist would determine if she met the criteria for either inpatient or outpatient commitment.

I wouldn't know where to begin. How would I feel about going to the city court to report my sister? What if they brought her to a hospital and the ED physician didn't agree to commit her? Would it destroy my relationship with my sister, creating the same kind of damage that occurred between Matthew and his parents? AOT is no doubt complicated for family members to initiate on their own. Clearly, what is needed are more AOT programs that involve a network of health care providers and judges, so that burden no longer falls solely on the family for keeping their loved ones in treatment and preventing tragic outcomes.

Another more collaborative legal option for individuals and their families who want to plan ahead for a mental health emergency is the psychiatric advance directive (PAD). These written agreements serve as a formal legal document in which a patient outlines what types of care or treatment they consent to or refuse if they become psychotic and lose touch with reality. It can also be an opportunity to write up what approaches have and have not worked in the past so that providers have a more complete history to inform care decisions. PADs allow patients to have a say in their treatment even if they're too ill to advocate for themselves in the moment—an approach that's gaining traction nationwide. The *New York Times* reports that "early research and experience suggest that PADs, authorized by law in twenty-seven states and possible in others as part of conventional medical advance directives, could help some of the millions of people with serious mental illness cope better and guide doctors treating them."[9]

Creating a PAD, which typically involves two forms, is something that an individual with SMI does when they are well. The first spells out treatment and care approaches while the second, a health care power of attorney form, temporarily grants a trusted loved one the authority to make decisions for an individual incapacitated by SMI. The necessary forms[10] are best filled out with legal assistance but can also be completed more informally. Unlike AOT, these forms are not court-ordered and may not be enforceable in every situation or jurisdiction, but they do provide an explicit record of an individual's wishes. What's so beautiful about this approach is that it creates not only a crisis plan, but a crisis *collaboration*. This is particularly important when dealing with people whose illnesses often render them alienated and marginalized.

Whether we like it or not, jails, judges, and law enforcement are already intimately involved in overseeing and managing mental health care, and it is critical to know how to leverage the law for treatment, not punishment. The new paths to "therapeutic jurisprudence" offer individuals and families more options for avoiding the revolving door of insufficient care.

CHAPTER 6

THE KINDNESS OF STRANGERS

I meet Debbie, a twenty-five-year-old Latina woman, as she lies strapped to a gurney in the LAC+USC psych ED. Thick black hair frames her open and earnest face as she calmly answers the questions of the admitting psychiatrist. "What are you seeing?" he asks.

"I'm seeing, like, a person with a jumpsuit," she replies.

He reviews her chart from a prior admission. "I read last year that you jumped out of a window and broke your leg. Why did you jump out of the window?"

"Because I felt like I was in danger and I thought I seen, like, this man and I thought he was gonna, like . . ." Debbie's voice trails off, and the doctor completes her sentence.

"Hurt you?"

"Yeah."

Then he asks about her wrist and the bruises on her arms. "Are those from your boyfriend?" Yes, she replies.

After the intake, I sit down with the psychiatrist who evaluated her. "She was hitting her boyfriend?"

"She attacked her boyfriend," he answers. "She was scratching him. She was assaultive to him and her family members, and she was just kind of out of control." He turns toward a computer screen that's lit up with an x-ray of Debbie's right wrist and moves the cursor along a fracture line in the bone. "You know, it's always amazing when the families report that the patient has been violent," he says. "She's been pretty calm with us."

"The intramuscular Ativan injection might've helped," I say.

Later, I ask Debbie what happened. "He hurt my feelings. I basically started whaling on him and then I smashed my hand. I basically wanted to hurt him." She struggles to explain how this altercation landed her in a psychiatric ED. "It just happens that way when you wanna be with somebody so bad but . . . You treat them really well and spend time with them, and after that you just wanna, like, always be there with them and you don't really try to hurt them, but, at the same time you just wanna protect them." And then, she continues haltingly, her face blank, her eyes wide, explaining how she started seeing things that aren't there. "I was seeing, basically, people that are from movies that would hurt people and you would think they are going to do it to you, but they're not."

I wonder what will happen next to Debbie. She's been on antipsychotic drugs before, and this is her third psych ED visit. Even if she's admitted, and hospital psychiatrists stabilize her symptoms, what then? What plan will they have in place, beyond a handful of pills and a paper informing her to follow up for an ongoing prescription, to keep her from another crisis that lands her back in the emergency room? Where will Debbie live if her family either can't or won't take her in? What kind of future lies ahead?

For the time being, Debbie is safe and relaxed. The ED is also, for a brief moment, remarkably calm. Two receptionists seated at computer stations behind safety glass take a breather. One pulls out her cell phone and hits play on Demarco's "I Love My Life," swaying in her chair. "I love my life. I love my life," the song begins. The woman beside her starts moving, too.

Debbie, wearing two hospital gowns, sipping from a flex straw in a foam cup, her right wrist wrapped in a cast, climbs off her gurney. She rocks side to side to the music, eyes closed, a smile on her face. From twenty feet away, one of the receptionists behind the Plexiglas watches. Debbie opens her eyes and meets her gaze. The two women smile at each other, both still swaying. Then the song—and the moment— ends. The receptionists return to their work—communicating with emergency dispatchers, calling for transport, and ushering patients into the ED—and Debbie returns to her gurney.

• • •

A year later, I meet up with Debbie and her boyfriend, Don, at a grassy park, where palm trees bend in the cold breeze overlooking the ocean. Shortly after she was discharged, she met Don, forty years her senior, at a donut shop. The former Marine, who uses a wheelchair, is disabled by multiple illnesses including diabetes and cardiovascular diseases. He was living alone at the time. Debbie, meanwhile, had been living on the streets. Don invited her to stay at his place until she got herself together. Between coughs and puffs on his e-cigarette, he tells me the story. "She helped me tremendously and got my house, my pets, everything in order so I realized at that time that she was a keeper, you know? So, we started hanging out more and more."

Debbie smiles. "We got to talking and he offered to help me and eventually, we just really, really connected," she says, giggling. "We try to help each other out and make sure that we're emotionally and physically stabilized and make sure that we're both loving each other as much as we can."

Over the year that they've been together, Debbie has managed to stay out of the hospital. "I don't hear any voices," she tells me. "I don't have any hallucinations. I'll get nightmares and those are not as vivid as they used to be." She's been getting a regular injection of an antipsychotic that lasts for a month and avoids the challenges of daily medication compliance. "It helps me sleep for the most part, because when I don't sleep I lose track of reality. It helps with my focusing and basically keeping my mental attitude at a good pace, and not sidetrack or think of other things, like, things that scare me, for example, loud noises or banging, stuff like that." But what has most helped her get better, she says, is "seeing the ocean and being with my fiancé. He always tells people that he feels that angels brought us together and—"

"I really do," interjects Don.

"I really, really feel like it's angels plus a higher power," Debbie finishes.

They show me their apartment and point out the ways in which they've have been crafting a life together—"like a start-up," Don says, as Debbie lays out his heart pills.

But another year later, when we catch up again, all is not wine and roses.

Debbie had wanted a normal life with Don, complete with a home, a wedding, and a baby. "For a long time that we've known each other we were trying to conceive because we were trying to get married and have the whole baby thing and have the whole honeymoon," she told me earlier. "We were going to take our camper, drive to the mountains, to the desert, wherever the breeze took us." But when she started feeling better she'd stopped getting her injections and began to free-fall. I can't say for sure what prompted Debbie to cease taking her medication—the bother of getting an injection, the stigma of taking a psychiatric drug, or the side effects, which include lethargy, dry mouth, weight gain, or feeling spacey, just to name a few.

Now their relationship is spiraling. I visit the day after a fight between them got so out of hand that neighbors called the police. Debbie has just returned to the apartment after sleeping on a friend's couch. Before long, the couple's conversation veers into fraught, clearly well-trod, territory: the pregnancy that Debbie insists she's carrying, and how she's been trying to make the home they have "suitable and healthy—not just to the minimum standards" for the baby's arrival.

"You sure you want to discuss this?" Don gives notice as I sit with them in the living room, but Debbie persists. Wearing a U.S. Marine Corps veteran cap, he leans back on the couch, legs crossed, smoking a Pall Mall. A tabletop fan blows a haze of smoke around the cluttered apartment, the ashtray perched on an upholstered ottoman beside a Marine Corps mug.

"I'm pretty much full term now," Debbie says, her voice cracking. She has put on weight since I saw her last—a side effect of her medication, probably—but she hardly looks nine months pregnant. "He's a real strong baby and I'm about to pop any day now. But now the baby is sensing that his dad doesn't want him. I told you like two days ago that that's what the baby's telling me," she says to Don, "that he's trying to connect to me that you don't want him."

Don rests his hand on his chin, his face blank. His eyes squint ever so slightly when she speaks. "How do I address that?" he asks, his voice measured. "How do I respond?"

"Do you have anything to believe in other than science?"

"There is no baby!" Don says, raising his voice slightly.

"Do you have any religion? Because when I met you, you did."

"Of course I do. Yeah. Of course I do," he replies. "How many doctors have told you there is *no* pregnancy? How many doctors have told you there's *no* baby in there? How many? There's got to be no less than five."

"You're going to see it with your own eyes. Why do they have to tell you?" Then she issues a threat: "You're not cutting any umbilical cord!"

Don turns to face her. "In all probability I'll have a baby before you do, so why don't you stop that shit, okay? There is no baby. You need to get on your medication. You need to get your head and ass wired together. Because all this other bullshit, it's funny, and I get a kick out of it sometimes, but now it's getting to be crazy, you know what I mean? Whether you're with me or not, you need that medication."

Debbie accuses Don of failing to be a protector, a father figure.

"I'm supposed to be the protector?" he asks. "There is no possible way for me to protect *you* from *you*. Can't do it. The only thing that's going to help you is your medication, get on a program. I have no confidence in this relationship," he says, finally. "There's nothing good here. No happy ending. It's just, this is what happens when people collide. They just have to split up because it's dangerous. It's a dangerous situation. I want to take a pass." He reaches for his pack of Pall Malls.

"There's no hall pass in this relationship, trust me," says Debbie, staring at him.

When I ask her where she'll spend the night, she says at her aunt's but that she can't stay there for long.

Don's tone softens a bit. "I think what you need to do is get your medication that you're supposed to get and then we can talk. Okay? I don't want to see you just go wandering the streets again."

But Debbie is already on her feet. "I don't want to talk to you. We're done. Everything that I've seen, I want you as far away from me as I can have you. I'm out of here."

"Then go. That's better for all of us," he says, a twisted, regretful look on his face. "Good luck to you."

Debbie pulls on a leather jacket, slings a small backpack over her shoulder, and heads for the door.

Outside she stands in the street, hands on her hips, biting her lip. "It's not hard for me, though," she says.

"What's not hard for you?" I ask.

"To accept that I'm homeless." She shakes her head and I watch her face shift from despair to resolve before a slight smile appears. She walks away, once again joining the ranks of the untold number of women with SMI who lack secure housing.

Compared with men who have the same psychiatric diseases (as well as with women in general), women who have schizophrenia, schizoaffective disorder, bipolar disorder, and major depression are more likely to be suicidal, to suffer from multiple medical conditions or substance abuse disorders (SUDs), and to die an early death.[1] Although both men and women with psychiatric diseases are at significant risk for crime victimization, women with SMI are almost twice as likely to have been beaten, sexually assaulted, or otherwise abused.[2] They are up to five times more likely than the general population to have been victims of sexual assault[3] and are more likely to wind up in jail.

Women with SMI are much more likely to be incarcerated than men with SMI, and the fastest-growing demographic in American prisons is women.[4] More than 65 percent of women in prison have a history of a mental health problem, and 32 percent of women in jail report having had serious psychological distress within the prior thirty days.[5] According to a 2018 U.S. Department of Housing and Urban Development count, women comprise 31 percent of the sheltered population and 27 percent of the unsheltered population.[6] SMI estimates among the female homeless population are limited, in part because most relevant research studies focus on men. However, the number of women experiencing homelessness has been increasing in recent years among both the sheltered and non-sheltered populations at rates up to three times that for men.[7]

Two years after they split, Don tells me he can't find Debbie. A family friend says she hasn't heard from her in years. Turning to the Internet, I finally spot her name on the public list of individuals incarcerated in the Los Angeles County Jail system.

The sheriff's department permits me to see Debbie on a Friday afternoon, outside normal visiting hours. I find my way into a large white building in an unpopulated wasteland of industrial complexes, where I lock my cell phone in a box with a key. As the deputies direct me through a series of steel doors to a holding area, I can hear screaming down the hallway. A few minutes later, Debbie appears, dressed in a yellow shirt and blue pants—the same Los Angeles Correctional Facility uniform that has been worn by all of the adults I have been following since first meeting them in the ED.

Debbie has put on perhaps fifty pounds, maybe more, since I saw her last—the same weight gain that I'd seen in Johanna and Monte over the years, side effects of their antipsychotic medications. She smiles at me broadly, and for a moment I am so taken by how happy I am to see her that I forget the shock of visiting her in this context. She takes her seat on the other side of the table, sitting square in her chair, seemingly at ease with her surroundings. A single handcuff chained to the tabletop is available for use with more violent individuals, but Debbie requires no restraint. Despite everything that has happened, she seems to be the same sweet soul I met four years earlier.

"How is it here?" I ask.

"Pretty good," she says, flashing the cherubic smile that I remember.

"Really?"

"It's not so bad, I like my bunkie."

Debbie fills in the blanks for me: a string of arrests, each resulting in a few months in jail. First, she was arrested for opening the birdcages at a pet store, believing she was Snow White, freeing the birds so they could return to the forest and be reunited with the dwarves. After her release, she broke into a neighbor's home and grabbed some money from the laundry room. The family she was robbing was standing right outside, and they quickly spotted her. She waited patiently for the police to arrive. That landed her in jail for another few months. After she got out, Debbie had to meet with a probation officer. When she failed to keep their appointments—which can be difficult when your psychosis leaves you disconnected from reality— she was rearrested for violating the terms of her release. Now she's been behind bars for four months while jail psychiatrists work to stabilize her mental health enough that she can appear in court.

Sitting in this cold concrete room, Debbie seems lucid and clearheaded, maintaining eye contact as we chat. But a beat later, she stares off in the distance. Her smile gets brighter, her eyes wider, and she begins talking *at* me instead of *to* me. That's when she says her father, who left her family when she was seven, is Tom Cruise, and that Johnny Depp is her boyfriend. She and Depp have sex once in a while, but they're on and off, and she doesn't know if she can take the fact that he's so unreliable. My heart sinks. The Debbie I recognized was there a moment before, but now she is lost in the stories she's weaving. She tells me her grandfather died many years ago, but he's just been playing dead in order to find her dad, who is also playing dead. I dare not ask about the baby she believed she was carrying, or her relationship with Don. I suspect that the Risperdal is managing the worst of her symptoms, such as agitation and hearing voices and seeing things, but she is clearly still ill.

When our time is up, Debbie tells me I have to exit first and that the guards will come for her after. I hate leaving her there. The deputy at the front desk motions me through one set of double doors to the next. The first set closes behind me. I hear a buzzer and push, but the door won't budge. The buzzer goes off again and I push, panic rising. Finally, I notice a sign that says, SLIDE, DON'T PUSH. I slide and escape. After retrieving my cell phone, I stop to use the men's room at the visitor's center before my long car ride. Water drips from the ceiling. All the urinals are full. I have to step through puddles to get reasonably close to one while water sprinkles my head.

Back in the fresh air, I turn to look at the concrete building, silent and foreboding as a tomb. For people who hear voices, what must those voices sound like in a place like this? Still, the uncomfortable truth is that Debbie seems happy, much happier than she was the last time I saw her. What does that say about how she feels about her life on the outside? And what lies ahead for her once she is out of jail?

When I get home to New York, I call Debbie's public defender in Los Angeles to follow up. It takes weeks to get him on the phone. Like most court-appointed attorneys, he has an overwhelming backlog of clients. When we reach each other, he proudly tells me that Debbie has been released. For four months, Debbie had been sitting in jail because, in the eyes of the law, her psychosis prevented her from assisting in her own defense. The medicines that the jail psychiatrist prescribed enabled Debbie to regain her sanity—just enough to meet the court's standards for competency. Her lawyer argued that now that she was better, she should be released with *time served*, meaning that Debbie had spent long enough in jail to pay for her crime of not showing up for a meeting with her probation officer. With that, she was "free," whatever that means for a homeless woman with chronic and often untreated psychosis who is again dependent on the kindness of strangers.

I felt like I was watching the exact scenario that Dr. Torrey had explained to me years earlier: "The problem is that the mentally ill end up in jail because they get arrested, mainly for petty crimes, and as a result they cycle in and out of the jails without ever getting any sustained and consistent treatment." After accruing a criminal record, many people with SMI become that much more unemployable, they get flung further down the dark downward trajectory of society's outcasts, and they become living examples of the futility of dealing with problems by locking people up.

Ultimately, where should Debbie be? No one wants to see a return to the nadir of mass institutionalization, but we can't neglect the reality that some people need long-term care. Instead, we must create compassionate care options that prioritize treatment over punishment. When a person with SMI is charged with a crime, interaction with the criminal justice system is unavoidable. In these cases, at least in jurisdictions where such a path exists, engagement with an MHC can offer an alternative to incarceration, motivating many people to get help who might not otherwise have done so. In MHCs, specially trained judges work with probation officers and mental health care providers to create a treatment and rehabilitation program for participant defendants. There are two basic varieties:

"pre-adjudication" programs, in which the defendant's criminal charge is held in abeyance with the promise of dismissal upon successful completion, and "post-adjudication" programs in which the defendant agrees to plead guilty and the reward for completion ranges from a suspended sentence to expungement. Under all models, the defendant agrees to plead guilty and follow the court-ordered plan, which can include therapy and medication for SMI and SUD, medication-compliance monitoring, substance-abuse testing, vocational training, and supervised housing. These programs allow judges to set expectations for the person's conduct and cooperation with a reasonable treatment plan. The period of required participation could be six months, a year, or more, with frequent court visits required throughout to allow the judge to monitor progress.[8] Although participation in an MHC is voluntary, choosing not to participate or failure to abide by the therapeutic requirements to comply with treatment can lead to jail time. The number of jurisdictions with an MHC option is expanding nationwide, bringing this opportunity to more and more people shuffled between the streets and the jails—including Monte.

• • •

Two years after his encounter with Nurse Practitioner Ellis in the Psych ED, Monte was arrested for breaking the window at a 7-Eleven while in the midst of a manic episode. He had gone off his medication. The cost of damages to the convenience store—more than $400—made his crime a felony, which meant a third "strike" on his record that would bring a mandatory three years in California state prison.

Monte walks into the courtroom in a fluorescent yellow shirt printed with the words LA COUNTY JAIL and sits quietly at a table, his hands behind his back in two sets of handcuffs linked together to accommodate his considerable size. His lawyer had argued, with Patrisse's prodding, that what Monte needs is a treatment bed, not a cell. Now the judge would issue his verdict.

He calls the court to order. "I've got a report about whether you would be a good candidate for this program. If you were to be placed into this program, it might do you some good. You're charged in count one with destruction of property with a value of more than $400. It's a felony. Do you understand the charge against you?"

"Yes, sir," Monte replies.

If the judge goes ahead, Monte will have to undergo mental health treatment for up to a year under the supervision of the Los Angeles Department of Mental Health. "It's going to be tighter supervision than ordinary probation, but if you're willing to do it we're willing to try and hook you up with the people who can give you help," the judge says.

Although the court rules in his favor, Monte remains in the Twin Towers of LA County Jail for four months until a treatment bed can be found. Patrisse tells me that her brother is a "gentle giant," but when the treatment centers interview him, they only see the "giant" part. Still, Monte is undoubtedly one of the lucky ones: because his case was heard by a judge who believes in the MHC approach, he is redirected from jail to treatment. Now he has a shot at reclaiming his health. And because he has a loyal support team, he is in much better stead than people like Debbie.

The idea of MHCs took off after drug courts, which were introduced in 1989, began to provide court-supervised, structured, community-based treatment for addiction.[9] Today the number of MHCs has grown from four jurisdictions in 1997 to more than

350, with programs in almost every state.[10] These programs reduce rates of re-arrest and re-incarceration among participants,[11] and even if they *are* re-arrested, participants tend to get charged with less serious crimes, and to go longer before re-offending, as well as being significantly less likely to commit violent acts than other detainees.[12] Although MHCs have become more prevalent in the last two decades, most people still don't know about them.

That a judge can dictate the terms of long-term medical care that can possibly involve involuntary institutionalization and the administration of mind-altering medicines with serious side effects is concerning, right? But like it or not, mandated treatment works. Monte's life is the best I've seen for him in the two years following his court-monitored treatment. With medication and talk therapy, he's even been able to keep a seasonal job selling Christmas trees. His employer tells me that Monte is never anything less than diligent, showing up every day with a smile. His recovery has not been easy, nor without its ups and downs, and Patrisse and her mother worry every day. They never forget that Monte remains just one strike away from prison, or one altercation with law enforcement away from a fatal outcome that has befallen many people with mental illness. For now, though, he is safe.

CHAPTER 7

EARLY AND EFFECTIVE INTERVENTION

"I'm a woman with chronic schizophrenia." That's how Professor Elyn Saks begins her TED Talk, which has been viewed more than 3.6 million times. "I have spent hundreds of days in psychiatric hospitals. I might have ended up spending my life in the back ward of a hospital, but that isn't how my life turned out."

To shed light on the experience of psychosis from the inside out, she recounts a story from her time as a student at Yale Law School. On a Friday night early in the term, she and two friends met up at the library for a study date. "But we didn't get far before I was talking in ways that made no sense," she recalls.

"Memos are visitations," she told them. "They make certain points. The point is on your head. Pat used to say that. Have you killed anyone?" Then she invited her friends to join her on the roof, where she began singing, loudly. When they asked her what was going on, she announced, "This is the real me," and continued singing: "Come to the Florida sunshine bush. Do you want to dance?"

Her friends asked if she was on drugs.

"No way, no drugs. Come to the Florida sunshine bush, where there are lemons, where they make demons." Frightened, her friends went inside. Eventually Saks made it to her dorm room, but she couldn't settle down. "My head was too full of noise, too full of orange trees and law memos I could not write and mass murders I knew I would be responsible for. Sitting on my bed, I rocked back and forth, moaning in fear and isolation."

This hadn't been the first time Saks had lost her brilliant mind to psychosis, nor would it be the last. Saks had a brief psychotic episode at age sixteen or seventeen, which her parents had inaccurately attributed to drug use. Then she had her first "official" psychotic break while studying at Oxford University at age twenty-one. As she describes in her memoir, *The Center Cannot Hold: My Journey through Madness*, her mental state had been deteriorating for weeks.

After a night spent lying "awake in a pool of sweat, unable to sleep, with a mantra running through [her] head: *I am a piece of shit and I deserve to die . . .*" she realized she was in danger. "The thoughts of death were all around me."[1] She admitted herself into a day program at a mental hospital that consisted of group therapy, individual sessions with a psychiatrist, board games, and stays in a living room–like "day room." Because she considered taking psychiatric drugs "cheating," she refused all medications. She felt she didn't deserve to consume the oxygen she breathed and decided that pouring gasoline over herself and lighting a match was the most "fitting end for a person as evil as I." The hospital staff insisted she needed inpatient care and Saks agreed to be admitted and begin taking antidepressants. The medication, along with therapy sessions with a doctor she trusted, helped quiet her suicidal thoughts, allowing her to return to her studies, at least for a time.

Saks readmitted herself eight months later. She had stopped eating or showering or doing laundry. She muttered to herself and gesticulated wildly and spent whole days rocking back and forth trying to soothe her addled mind and gaunt, agitated body. She heard commands that ordered her to burn her flesh, which she did with cigarettes, lighters, electric heaters, and boiling water. Although her doctors and the staff were aware she was self-harming, Saks never revealed that the impetus for her self-destructive behavior was a "commanding impulse" that "came from inside my head but was not mine." She feared their laughter. "As frightened as I was, the thought of derision frightened me even more. It was a life-threatening deception, somewhat along the lines of hiding recurrent chest pains from one's cardiologist from embarrassment." It's hard to imagine a clearer demonstration of the deadly consequences of the stigma surrounding mental illnesses such as schizophrenia.

Several months later, Saks was discharged again, stabilized but with an official prognosis of "very poor." Despite this bleak pronouncement, her later hospitalization while at Yale, and other mental health crises, she has maintained a full life and a superlative career with the help of medication and psychotherapy. She earned a master's degree at Oxford, graduated from Yale Law School, and today is a distinguished professor of law psychology and psychiatry at the University of Southern California's law school. She has also gained tremendous insight into the workings of her own mind.

"I think it's a myth that people with mental health disorders can't do the things that most people do and value doing, like work, having relationships, getting married, having children, that kind of thing," she tells me. As a highly successful person who speaks openly about her experiences, she is helping to dismantle the stereotype that people with SMI, particularly schizophrenia, are doomed to live thwarted, isolated lives.

Unlike many of the people I met in the psych ED, Professor Saks didn't spend decades languishing in jails or on the streets. She didn't self-medicate with street drugs. She was neither poor nor uneducated. She wasn't tied down to a cot in a jail cell. After years of attentive care, Professor Saks accepted the chronic nature of her diagnosis, acquiesced to her need for antipsychotic medication, and found a regimen that would keep her symptoms on a low enough simmer to allow her to survive and thrive. Although she is by no means "cured," Saks's biography offers evidence that relatively early, consistent intervention can turn the tide even for the most aggressive cases.

Just as a cancer diagnosis at stage one versus stage three offers hope for better outcomes, early intervention in cases of SMI is critical. "It is very clear that the longer someone goes untreated the worse, on average, their long-term prognosis," Dr. Goff, director of the Nathan Kline Institute for Psychiatric Research, tells me. There's also a tendency "for some people, with each relapse, to never quite regain their previous level of symptom control."

Steven Adelsheim, MD, director of the Stanford Center for Youth Mental Health and Wellbeing in the Department of Psychiatry, says something similar: "Like other medical conditions, the longer an issue goes on untreated, the more serious and severe the symptoms can be." Once the illness has progressed, it can be difficult for even aggressive treatment to change its course;[2] on the flip side, the sooner someone starts on antipsychotic medications, the more likely they are to get well.[3] This raises the question: Why does a longer duration of untreated illness (DUP) make a disease such as schizophrenia or mania more destructive and harder to get under control? It's no exaggeration to say that untreated psychosis is actually toxic to the brain (neurotoxicity), as overactive brain systems destroy cerebral matter, with excess dopamine, catecholamine, and stress hormones seen as potential bad actors.[4]

For some people, untreated psychosis for extended periods is correlated with loss of brain volume, too, particularly in the memory center called the hippocampus and the reasoning centers in the frontal lobes.[5] These effects seem to be cumulative, meaning that it's not only the initial psychosis that affects the brain but subsequent episodes that are often caused when people stop their medication and relapse. However, we don't reliably see evidence of this neurotoxicity on brain scans, and only a small minority of people with psychosis have an identifiable organic abnormality. Whether these cumulative effects have to do with neurological changes, learned bad habits, or simply the fallout from long-term hopelessness remains to be seen.

What is clear is that it pays to focus on taking early action. Practically speaking, however, early intervention rarely happens. First, proper diagnosis can take years, since it relies on the progression of symptoms over time; just because someone has had a psychotic *episode* does not mean they have a psychotic *disorder*. Similarly, episodes of severe depression may not be recognized as part of bipolar disorder until mania manifests repeatedly as well, which can take years after the first symptoms come to the fore. It takes time, as we say in medicine, to reveal what the true illness is.

Another problem is acceptance. These are not diagnoses that most people come to accept easily. Individuals and their families alike often resist, with good reason, being branded with a serious mental disorder. Given the deep-rooted stigma and sense of despair surrounding these diseases, coping with such a diagnosis is a lot like dealing with a terminal physical illness, including a whole lot of bargaining and denial that precedes acceptance. Unfortunately, a prolonged grief cycle can postpone any effective action that might arrest the disease process.

The third problem comes with identifying and implementing an appropriate course of treatment. Care recommendations change based on symptoms. When bipolar disorder is first diagnosed as depression, for example, proper medications may not be prescribed until the illness reveals itself years down the line.

Saks faced each of these hindrances to early intervention. Initially hesitant to take medications, she relied on psychotherapy, which ultimately proved insufficient to manage the escalation of her disease. Even when she did agree to medication, the antidepressant she was given was not the proper drug to stave off psychosis. For years she fought against the label and the implications of schizophrenia, repeatedly going off the antipsychotics she had been prescribed. "I felt that if I could manage without medication, I could prove that, after all, I wasn't really mentally ill; it was some terrible mistake," she explains in her TED Talk. "My motto was the less medicine, the less defective."

While she was teaching at the University of Southern California law school, during one of the thirty or forty times she attempted to go off medication over the course of a decade, she tried again to ditch the drugs. Psychosis took over, leaving her "writhing in agony" convinced that "evil beings poised with daggers" would "slice me up in thin slices or make me swallow hot coals." It took the coaxing of trusted psychiatrists, friends, and family for Saks to realize that she "could no longer deny the truth, and I could not change it. The wall that kept me, Elyn, Professor Saks, separate from that insane woman hospitalized in years past, lay smashed and in ruins." Accepting her diagnosis and committing to rigorous treatment ("four- to five-day-a-week psychodynamic psychotherapy for decades and continuing, and excellent psychopharmacology") has made all the difference, as have the supportive relationships in her life, both personal and collegial.

One more element that can hinder early intervention is a sometimes-unwelcoming medical approach that can include restraints. Saks says that she was fortunate to receive her first treatment for SMI in the UK, which employs a markedly different approach to care:

> In England, treatment recommendations were always just that—recommendations. To leave a hospital, to stay in it, to take medications, to participate in group activities or not—they never forced any of it on me, and each time the decision was mine. Even at my craziest, I interpreted this as a demonstration of respect. When you're really crazy, respect is like a lifeline someone's throwing you. Catch this and maybe you won't drown.

Saks was never restrained, even when she was most actively harming herself with burns. Had she been in the United States at the time, the American approach might well have turned her off from ever seeking help again.

While at Yale Law School, Saks discovered firsthand the difference between the two countries. Following her ill-fated study date in the library, she wound up in an emergency room where psychiatrists failed to convince her to relinquish the six-inch nail that she gripped in her pocket as protection from the people who were trying to kill her. Finally, a doctor pried the nail away and a team of what she called "ER goons" pounced. They slammed her down onto a bed with such force that she "saw stars." Then they bound her arms and legs with thick leather straps and forced her to swallow a bitter liquid. "Strapped down, unable to move, and doped up, I can feel myself slipping away," she wrote in her memoir. "I am finally powerless. I am like a bug, impaled on a pin, wriggling helplessly while someone contemplates tearing my head off." She had nightmares for years.

I asked Saks if being restrained affected her attitude about seeking help. "Absolutely," she replied. "It deterred me from ever going to an ER again, which I'm glad I never did. It might have been useful, at times, to be able to get some care when I was really struggling, but the idea of being tied [up] again was just so horrible and traumatic that I would never, ever dream of doing it."

While writing a paper about the ethics of the practice, Saks asked an eminent psychiatrist, "'Don't you think that restraints must be very degrading and painful?' He said, 'Oh, you don't understand, Elyn. *These* people are psychotic. They're different from you and me, and they don't experience restraints the way we would.' I did not have the courage, in that moment, to tell him, 'No. *We're* not different. It's very traumatic for us, too.'"

Perhaps restraints are a telling symbol of the general lack of respect and hostility our society shows people who have mental illness. We often treat them as the "other," devoid of humanity or any identity beyond their SMI—summarizing the entirety of their mind as "sick."

As a psychiatrist, I see that the same mental traits can lead to various kinds of mental illnesses, or extraordinary professional achievements, or both. The same traits that make you unusually empathic and tuned into the feelings of others in an intimate relationship can make you overly sensitive and painfully fearful of criticism. The same personality traits of confidence and dogged self-determination that enable you to succeed in your business affairs can make you egocentric and arrogant with others in your personal life. Among great artists, we see often that the border between their genius and their madness is permeable. There are many examples of extremely successful people who use their brain differences for fame and fortune only to pass on their genes to their children who develop devastating mental illnesses. To me this suggests that extreme brain differences can be a blessing or a curse. Hence, there is a more accurate, less pathological, and less judgmental way of describing brain differences.

The term *neurodiversity* characterizes variations in the brain as the result of human heterogeneity. Some mental health advocates see this framing—which has already shaped a burgeoning movement around autism, dyslexia, and other neurological conditions, categorizing them as natural variances rather than pathologies or disorders—as the next wave in activism.[6] Neurodiversity says that each of us possesses a unique brain with special sensitivities and abilities that can be *assets* as well as deficits. This perspective highlights the gifts and skills associated with some brain anomalies. It gets us to think about our "abnormalities" as potential advantages in the right circumstances.

I've seen this concept misused to justify a denial of mental illness altogether, but as a psychiatrist, I also see how this approach welcomes people with different minds into the conversation and helps people with SMI to realize that they are multifaceted, not just sick. It has never once been productive to disparage someone just because they are outside the "norm."

One thing that became eminently clear to me as I spoke with Saks was that she has an extraordinary brain. No doubt brilliant, she also struck me as unusually perceptive. She has uncommon sensitivities along with a remarkable capacity for explaining the inner workings of her own mind. As I learned more about her experiences and read her descriptions of her inner landscape, I could understand how, under stress, that profound sensitivity might transform perceptions into piercing intrusions. It also became clear that Saks is not an extraordinary observer *despite* her schizophrenia. Instead, her keen awareness no doubt feeds both her scholarship and the empathy that makes her an extraordinary teacher.

Professor Saks is less sanguine. She tells me, "It's really cool that some people can understand what they're going through as something different and, maybe, an asset in some ways rather than just a terrible problem," but "I tend to think of it as a terrible problem." If there were a pill that could cure her once and for all, she would take it without hesitation.

• • •

Professor Saks may not have been fully treated at the onset of her illness, but she certainly found more collaborative care and at an earlier point than many of the people I've met in my research. Dr. Adelsheim has spent many years developing early detection and intervention programs to address depression, anxiety, and prodromal symptoms of psychosis,[7] as well as first episodes of the disease. To surmount the hurdles of stigma and misinformation, he is also working on creating community-based websites "designed and marketed directly to young people." He explains it this way:

> What we're really targeting is easy access for twelve- to twenty-five-year-olds to come in and get early mental health care, primary care, supported education deployment, early addiction treatment, [and] early psychosis programs so that young people . . . might feel comfortable coming in when they're dealing with these early anxiety or other kinds of symptoms and can be

followed. And if they start to move toward having psychotic symptoms, the co-locator of the early psychosis program is also there to be able to do a warm handoff for that young person and family to access the family support and the early treatments.

Psychosocial treatments are a crucial first course of action. Psychotherapy, exercise, good nutrition, and stress reduction are evidence-based approaches with few downsides. It also helps to avoid recreational drugs and substances that can harm the brain. Family education, too, can make a world of difference, especially if family members heed the advice of the experts who have documented that learning about psychiatric illnesses significantly improves outcomes for their loved ones and allows everyone to keep the faith.[8]

Hope is at the core of Dr. Dixon's work with OnTrackNY. The New York–based program, which she designed and oversees, helps young people showing early signs of mental illness to achieve their goals in school, work, and relationships. Participants work with a comprehensive team of clinicians, education, and employment specialists, including peer consultants who also have SMI, to find a job or complete school. The goal is to keep the lives of participants, ages sixteen to thirty, from getting derailed by their disease.

. Just as important as the practical services that OnTrackNY provides is the attitude with which the team delivers them. "If we had not a single new drug, not a single new psychosocial treatment, if we simply offered what we have and we offered it in a frame that was positive and hopeful, and didn't tell people from the day they entered the program that they're going to lead a life of disability—and it's not like they say that directly—what would it look like? How would things change? I think that they would change for the better."

Dr. Dixon reminded me that when she and I began our training in the 1980s, the very *definition* of schizophrenia included a deteriorating course. In fact, if a patient did well—finished school, had a job, had a sustained romantic relationship, and raised a family—our professors would claim the diagnosis had been wrong. Back then, schizophrenia meant only doom. "I know that I've always done better when someone says that they believe in me," explains Dr. Dixon. "Why would a person with mental illness be any different than that?"

With early interventions, patient and family education, and support, leading a productive life is possible for most people diagnosed with an SMI. Like other successful programs, OnTrackNY actively involves participants in designing their own treatment and recovery and aims to preserve their dignity and self-determination above all. Its focus on open dialogue is our best hope for changing our culture of denial, shame, and ignorance—a culture that abetted my sister's decline and ultimate demise. Dr. Dixon, too, cites her own brother as an example of someone who might have done much better had he been treated earlier.

Maintaining an open dialogue about the realities of psychiatric illnesses alongside a healthy sense of optimism is at least half the battle. The other half is advancing our meager scientific understanding of these conditions.

• • •

One promising area of research on detection and intervention focuses on identifying early signs of illness among at-risk teenagers and young adults, between ages twelve and twenty-one. Tyrone Cannon, PhD, professor of psychology and psychiatry at Yale, studies the brain mechanisms that precede psychotic hallucinations and delusions, which he describes as "altered perceptions and be-liefs about the world and one's perceptions that are sort of at odds with the rest of the world." Dr. Cannon follows young people with recently altered thought and perception, like a feeling that their mind is playing tricks on them. They may describe a sense that ev-erything that used to be familiar "now seems strange or ominous," Dr. Cannon explains. "There's this sort of generalized feeling that something is different. Time is different, the world seems different in some way." This can lead to a low-grade suspiciousness, but with-out a specific notion of who or what has it in for them. Other amor-phous symptoms may include garbled noises, rather than the voices generally associated with a psychotic break.[9] They know that the noises are probably coming from inside their own head (whereas during true psychosis, the afflicted person believes that the voices are "real" and coming from an outside source).

Approximately 20 percent of young people experiencing these and similar symptoms, who are clinically deemed high-risk, pro-gress to a fully psychotic state within two years.[10] Of the 80 percent who don't, about one third continues to have the same low-intensity symptoms, another third shows some improvement, and the final third functionally recovers. The question becomes, what distin-guishes these different categories, particularly those in the unlucky 20 percent?

Carrie Bearden, PhD, professor of psychiatry and biobehavioral sciences and psychology at UCLA, researches progressions in bipo-lar disorder. The symptoms experienced by the adolescents and young adults she studies tend to be lower-grade manifestations of the full-blown disease, including milder forms of grandiosity, exag-gerated changes in mood or affect in quick succession, and sleep disruption. These at-risk young people may be impulsive risk-takers and/or may have attention deficit/hyperactivity disorder (ADHD). Dr. Bearden says roughly 5 percent of these youth go on to develop bipolar disorder within three years of their diagnosis of being at "clinical high risk for psychosis."

In an effort to predict who will get sick and why, researchers like Cannon and Bearden are working to identify physiological indicators of illness, including biomarkers. As a young doctor, I remember being forced to memorize the diagnostic labels in the *DSM III*—the latest bible of mental illness at the time. I quoted the diagnoses like an evangelical quotes the scriptures, knowing all the while that these categorizations were crude and the *DSM* is always in flux. Most psychiatrists would prefer if diagnoses were not solely phenomenological—determined by clusters of symptoms such as hearing voices or depressed mood—but instead based on biological markers such as brain scans, blood tests, or genetic chromosomal studies. Those kinds of organic manifestations would offer invaluable information to aid proper diagnosis, prevention, early detection, and treatment.

For example, brain scans reveal that many people who become— but are not yet—psychotic show abnormal patterns of communication between certain areas of the brain, with some structures overconnecting while others underconnect. Another possible biomarker is the stress hormone cortisol, which can be measured in saliva. Bearden's preliminary research has shown that "having higher cortisol levels in saliva was predictive of conversion to psychosis."[11]

Cannon's focus, at least recently, has been on identifying "factors that change dynamically as the symptoms worsen" because "they have a better chance of explaining *why* the symptoms are getting worse." In particular, he is trying to understand *progressive cortical thinning.* "There's a tendency in normal adolescent brain development for synapses to be pruned," he explains. This pruning is the standard mechanism through which the typical adolescent brain achieves adult capabilities by increasing efficiency in the cortex. Infants and young children need maximum power to acquire information about the world, and as a child's brain grows it forms synaptic connections through memories created and lessons learned. As we age, however, we become specialists. Trimming unused synapses helps strengthen the most important connections in the development of an adult brain. Think of it as a form of spring cleaning during which the brain gets rid of unused connections and thereby becomes more efficient.

Recently, researchers have discovered that *overly aggressive* pruning could be associated with the development of psychotic disease in adolescence and early adulthood.[12] Longitudinal study of structural MRIs now suggests what Bearden describes as "a steeper rate of gray matter loss in those who converted to a psychotic disorder" that scientists think may represent "an overly aggressive synaptic pruning process in those who develop psychosis." But Bearden explains, "there is no way to directly measure synaptic pruning in living humans." In other words, the data is interesting, but has not yet translated into anything that a doctor can use for diagnosis and treatment.

Cannon explains that among "clinical high-risk cases who develop psychosis, the rate of thinning in parts of the brain that are relevant to psychotic illnesses, including various parts of the prefrontal cortex, show an exaggerated rate of thinning." This, he says, not only is visible in sequential MRI scans but also seems to be confirmed by postmortem data on people with schizophrenia that reveals the nature of the cellular pathology.

At this point in my conversation with Cannon I had to ask what he thought all this might mean for future diagnoses. "Might we reach the point when a young person showing these early symptoms can get an MRI and the doctor will say, 'Ah, thinning cortex. Start the anti-psychotic today'?" But, of course, things are not that simple.

The first problem, he explains, is that the imaging data of brain alterations is not yet sophisticated enough to predict who will develop an SMI. Second, we can't forget that antipsychotics are not curative. "They don't arrest the underlying mechanisms of psychosis" but instead "put a damper on how invasive the psychotic material is into the consciousness of the patient." In other words, they don't stop or reverse the disease, just ease the symptoms. Third, the side effects of antipsychotics, as we've seen, can be enormously damaging in and of themselves. As a result, "people who work in this phase of illness in this population are for the most part not strong advocates of the use of antipsychotics until the person has developed full symptoms."

Although we are not yet able to reliably evaluate the rate of pruning or the thinness of the cortex as predictors of mental illness, these findings have encouraged researchers to take a closer look at possible causes of excessive pruning. Early findings from Beth Stevens, PhD, and Steven A. McCarroll, PhD, at Harvard suggest that it may be controlled by a part of our genes related to our immune reactions called the major histocompatibility complex, with a miscommunication of the immune system triggering the overzealous trimming.[13]

Other studies have found that deletions on certain areas of the genome are associated with a twenty-five-fold increase in the likelihood of developing schizophrenia.[14] Still others have corroborated a long-standing suspicion that overactivation of the dopamine system is correlated with psychosis.[15] (We have known since the 1950s about the connection between dopamine and psychosis, since anti-psychotics often work by exerting an antidopamine effect.)

Yet, as with all research concerning SMI, these findings are merely suggestive, and we remain years away from translating them into something that will benefit most patients. Moreover, biology is but one part of the cause. Under psychiatry's bio-psycho-social model, we believe that our brains exist in a dynamic flux with our psychology and the influence of our society and surroundings— each part of the triad in a constant push-pull with the other two. In time, I hope that we will find preventative medications that can be safely used with the earliest signs of SMI. But we're not there yet.

• • •

The painful irony of all the recent research supporting the efficacy of early intervention is the paucity of resources available for our youngest patients. The discussion of early intervention never seemed so pressing as one Friday night in 2013. The LAC+USC psych ED is filled—overfilled—with children. So many families have arrived with minors threatening violence or self-harm and displaying other disturbing behavior that Dr. Dias has cleared a regular pediatric ED waiting room to create a makeshift way station. Los Angeles County's ten total psych beds available to uninsured minors are already filled when twelve new patients arrive seeking help.

Eleven-year-old Delilah and her mother, Gloria, are among those waiting. That day, her teacher found a note. Delilah had written: "All day I have been feeling sad and thinking of suicide and running away from home. I would choke myself, drown myself, or use drugs to hurt myself." She's being bullied at her majority-Latino school because although her mother is Latina, her father is African American. He left when she was a baby, and Delilah feels his absence keenly. Depression such as Delilah's may not be as incapacitating and intractable as the psychosis of schizophrenia that hits a young adult in their early twenties, but it's no less deadly; suicide is the second-leading cause of death among people age fifteen to thirty-four,[16] and Dr. Dias takes her threats and previous attempt seriously. But she is not admitted, partly because Dr. Dias thinks her mother will be able to manage her symptoms at home, and partly because the nearest available hospital bed is more than a hundred miles away.

Seven-year-old Nick, an African American boy with wide eyes, long lashes, and closely cropped hair, is waiting, too. He lies in a gurney wearing blue pajamas decorated with cartoon animals that the hospital has provided, a white blanket pulled up to his chest. His mother is curled up beside him, stroking his face. To conduct their intake in private, Dr. Dias has to enlist the nurses to move another patient from the shared room.

Pulling up a chair and lowering the bed's safety rail so they can face each other, Dr. Dias asks Nick, "Can you tell us where you're at right now?"

"The hospital."

"Do you know why you're in the hospital?

"Because I cut myself." Nick's mother, her face inches from her son's, doesn't take her eyes off him.

"You cut yourself. What did you cut yourself with?"

"With scissors." Nick picks at his fingers, his voice quiet and wary.

"Scissors. What made you do that?"

"'Cause I got mad."

"And what made you mad?"

"When somebody just told my friend to stop playing with me, I just got a little bit mad."

"Can I see where you got cut?" asks Dr. Dias. The boy sits up and pulls aside the blanket. "Let's take a look." At school that day, the second grader had scratched an opening in his skin just below his knee. But the wound has already scabbed over and is small enough that it doesn't require a bandage. "Oh, my goodness. You actually really did cut yourself."

Nick answers Dr. Dias's questions. No, he hasn't cut himself anywhere else. No, he never cut himself before. Then Dr. Dias asks, "What made you take the scissors and cut your leg? What were you trying to do?"

"I was trying to calm down," explains Nick. "It makes me calm down."

His mother waits patiently, permitting Nick the space to speak for himself. But when the doctor addresses her directly she fills in the blanks. "He's talked about killing hisself and I've never heard it," she says. "I've heard it from other people. And the school found a note that he wrote." At that time, the school had called Child Protective Services, but ultimately, she says, "they just ignored it." She shakes her head in frustration. It's difficult to know what's going on with her son because he's so quiet. "He's very shy and he just suppresses his feelings deep inside, so it's hard to know when he's hurting or anything happens to him. But I do know he talks about death a lot." That started when he and his eight-year-old brother returned from living with his dad in Alabama for two years after she was laid off. "A lot of mental, verbal, and physical abuse happened," she says.

Prompted by Dr. Dias, Nick shares the details. "I'd get in trouble for crazy stuff," he says. "When I spilled milk at the store he slapped me in the back of my head and when I'd get home he'd whup me." His father used a belt that left marks on his body.

"And what else would he do?"

"He'd make me stand in the corner on one leg and if I fall off the leg, he'd whup me." Nick's wide eyes are wet but no tears fall.

"That sounds horrible. I'm really sorry to hear that you had to go through stuff that was that bad."

At the end of their conversation, when Dr. Dias asks what Nick needs help with, the boy says, "My anger problems." Then he asks Nick what three wishes he'd like granted. "The first one would be that my dad would be nicer to me. The second one would be that I stop . . . I stop . . . I stop getting mad and saying stuff like 'I want to kill myself.' And my third wish will be that I never get messed with again."

"Wow. Those are great wishes," says Dr. Dias. "I'm going to ask you one other question. If you could be any animal in the world, what animal would you be and why?"

"A zebra."

"Why would you be a zebra?"

"Because zebras, they're one of the nicer animals on the planet. They don't bite. And zebras, they have beautiful color and they're just nice. And they don't bite. They don't kill."

By the end of their chat, Dr. Dias has decided the boy will benefit from a few days in the hospital. "Think of it kind of like a vacation," he says, in a place "where nobody really knows you and you can start off fresh and clean. And I want you to talk about all the things you've been scared to talk about."

Nick's mom agrees with the doctor's prescription. "I want my son to get help," she says. The trouble is, there's no treatment bed in all of Los Angeles County available for him—or for the other kids in crisis.

Seventeen-year-old Sofia is also waiting. Ever since she told her parents several months ago about the sexual abuse she endured at the hands of her uncle at age five, she has been thinking about suicide every night. Last night, she tells the ED psychiatrist, she imagined swimming in the open ocean until her muscles shut down, "until my body tells me it's over, and I can't swim back." She imagined drowning and "then my body rests in the ocean." Her mind churned until she finally dozed off, before waking only a short time later. "So, you're waking up in the night," the doctor says. "Do you dream?"

"I don't dream. I have nightmares." In her nightmares, she's a small child trying to escape, to hide. "I'd just run everywhere, and there's no escape. Just trying to wake up, and I can't. So I feel my heart beating, and I just give up." Her sleeplessness has been leading her to doze off in class and her grades have begun to slip. She only finds solace in training to run marathons. "I run for new, open doors to see what I could find in other places, so I can be escaping where I have been."

"When you're running, do you think about the things that have happened to you?"

"I try not to," Sofia replies. "I notice my breathing. I notice my pace."

Again, the psychiatrist concludes that a hospital is the safest place for her. "I'm really glad that you came in," he says, "because I'm really glad that maybe we can step in and give you some assistance."

As director of a seriously overextended psychiatric ED, Dr. Dias is doing his utmost to provide the best possible care with limited resources. But nights like this leave him lamenting our society's abandonment of children in need. "The most vulnerable of our population, who are afflicted with mental illness at a very high rate and are in continuous need of acute psychiatric services for various reasons, don't have enough inpatient beds in the County of Los Angeles," he says.

Los Angeles is not alone. In fact, thanks to the County Department of Health Services, LAC+USC Medical Center is a last refuge for many. Mental health professionals, city officials, and advocates warn of the disastrous consequences of too few beds for young people nationwide. In Massachusetts in 2018, officials counted 155 patients in mental health crisis, many of them children, who had spent at least four consecutive days in an emergency room between February and May of that year. Several slept in the ED for two weeks while many others waited two or three days for a bed. Most were not permitted to go outside or leave their rooms, even to shower.[17]

When it comes to children, the stakes couldn't be higher. It is estimated that half of mental illnesses begin by age fourteen and three quarters by age twenty-four. While one in five children ages thirteen to eighteen has, or will develop, a mental illness, just over half of them receive specialized treatment,[18] and the often very long delays between the onset of symptoms and treatment—which can span decades—has significant consequences. The fact that most mental disorders begin in childhood and adolescence highlights that we must shift our focus to understanding the magnitude, risk factors, and progression of these illnesses. Yet both systemic and social barriers stand in the way of crucial research, facility access, and proper treatment.

When it is done well, however, treatment can be lifesaving. Delilah, who was sent back home after expressing suicidal thoughts, exemplifies what's possible, although her journey has never followed a straight path. Several months after her ED visit, she tells me she "was still emotionally unstable." Her problems at school worsened. "I didn't know how to cope with them, and I wasn't getting the help I needed." She found herself again in crisis, struggling with anxiety and depression. She told the school nurse that she had swallowed twelve Advil gel capsules to try to kill herself. (She thought that would be enough.) This time, her mother permitted her transfer to Bakersfield Behavioral Healthcare Hospital, the closest facility with available juvenile beds, 163 miles away from her home.

At first, Delilah wondered what she'd gotten herself into: "I saw a seven-year-old kid. He was there for trying to kill his mom." They took away her shoelaces. But the next morning at breakfast, it started to feel like a getaway. "You get to think about the things you've done," she says, and to ponder, "What is life?" The activities she participated in during her weeklong stay helped her reflect on the reasons she was in the hospital. "It was really worth it," she explains. "I actually left with a good memory from there." She also left with a treatment plan that included medication and psychotherapy. Three years later, she says that her hospitalization saved her life.

CHAPTER 8

STRENGTH IN (SMALL) NUMBERS, OR AMERICA IS WAKING UP

Spending on research for mental illness remains disproportionately low relative to its impact on society. By way of contrast, spending on breast cancer and HIV/AIDS research is much higher because of strong advocacy and political pressure. A mother whose son has SMI asked me, "Why is this okay? Where is the outrage? The ribbons, the races, and the ice bucket challenges?"

Reflecting our neglect, funding pools are lopsided, and not in SMI research's favor. Schizophrenia is one of the costliest diseases of our time, with an estimated annual social and economic cost of $155.7 billion,[1] but in 2019, SMI received about $452 million *total* in NIH research dollars, while cancer got $6 billion and heart disease more than $1 billion.[2] This despite projections that the global cost burden of mental illness may exceed that of cancer, cardiac disease, and all noncommunicable diseases for the more than one billion people with a mental disorder.[3] The section of NIH that funds mental health is NIMH, and its director, Josh Gordon, MD, laments that our understanding of mental illness is not yet at the point of identifying novel treatments. "We're trying to do a better job of figuring out who's at risk earlier, getting them into care earlier, and then testing interventions in that early time period that might delay the onset of psychosis, for example, or that might reduce the impact of the first episode," he tells me. "There just aren't the scientific opportunities. We could do more if we had more money."

In the meantime, families wait. A lot of families. Approximately 300 million people globally have depression, while 23 million people have schizophrenia and about 60 million have bipolar disorder.[4] According to a 2018 Lancet Commission report, mental illness is on the rise in every nation in the world and could cost the global economy up to $16 trillion between 2010 and 2030. This includes not only direct costs of health care but also productivity loss, as well as the incumbent costs of "social welfare, education, and law and order." In the United States, SMI costs $193.2 billion annually in lost earnings.[5] Meanwhile, less than half (42.6 percent) of American adults with psychiatric disorders received mental health care. For people with serious conditions, that number is 66.7 percent,[6] leaving a significant number of seriously ill people untreated.

So, where do they wait?

• • •

Jonathan Sherin, MD, PhD, director of the Los Angeles County Department of Mental Health, doesn't mince words. He says we didn't get rid of asylums in Los Angeles in the 1960s with deinstitutionalization; we just substituted the local asylum for an "indoor" one called the Los Angeles County Jail and an "outdoor" asylum called skid row. John Snook, director of the Treatment Advocacy Center, agreed that the dismantling of the asylum was really "transinstitutionalization"—transferring the care of patients from asylums to streets and prisons. We still hospitalize people, but they're "micro-hospitalizations," says Snook, referring to the average length of a U.S. psych hospital stay of three to five days.[7]

What Dr. Sherin, Snook, and many policy experts hold partly responsible for the mess is the IMD exclusion rule, enacted in 1965 as part of the Medicaid and Medicare legislation. Spearheaded by President Lyndon Johnson through amendments to the Social Security Act, the exclusion explicitly prohibited Medicaid from paying for patient care in state or private hospitals that specialize in mental health care.[8] The rationale was to disincentivize the founding of any new asylums or large psychiatric institutions funded with federal money.

In a 2019 issue of *Psychiatric Services* that presented both sides of the IMD exclusion debate, editors Dr. Dixon and Dr. Goldman explain that the rule "prohibits federal Medicaid payments for services delivered to individuals aged twenty-two to sixty-four years residing in IMDs," defined as "hospitals, nursing homes, or other institutions with more than sixteen beds that are primarily engaged in providing diagnosis, treatment, or care of persons with 'mental diseases' other than dementia or intellectual disabilities."[9] To repeat—no mental hospital with more than sixteen beds.

The IMD debate to permit larger mental hospitals stirs up fears that we will return to the nadir of mass institutionalization in huge asylums. In their 2015 paper, "Improving Long-Term Psychiatric Care: Bring Back the Asylum," Dominic A. Sisti and his colleagues conclude that inpatient facilities are an essential part of any successful strategy for improving the circumstances of people with SMI—"a necessary but not sufficient component of a reformed spectrum of psychiatric services." They remind us that there is a profound shortage of inpatient beds (just fourteen for every 100,000 people in the United States, a 95 percent decline from the 1950s).[10]

"Asylums never went away, they just grew into two varieties: posh for the wealthy (in the form of a handful of fancy $100,000-plus a year mental institutions) and prisons for the poor," says Cheryl Roberts, executive director of the Greenburger Center for Social and Criminal Justice. Roberts wants to establish "a new set of 'institutions,' defined broadly to include community outpatient clinics, residential inpatient facilities, and options in between." She also wants Medicaid funding for larger residential, nonhospital settings, often referred to as congregate care facilities, where people can receive longer-term, humane treatment and avoid ending up in a prison or jail bed. This would require amending the "so-called IMD exclusion in the Medicaid law that deprives poor Americans of the right to mental health care." (By the way, although federally funded hospitals can't have more than sixteen psych beds without special exceptions, there is no limit on the number of psych beds in prisons or jails. Just one tower of the Los Angeles County Jail contains roughly 1,500 beds filled with men with mental illness.)

Supporters of retaining the exclusion, like Jennifer Mathis, JD, at the Judge David L. Bazelon Center for Mental Health Law, question whether its impact has actually been negative at all. In *Psychiatric Services*, Mathis argued that "neither the IMD rule nor insufficient hospital beds is the primary problem."[11] Instead, she cited the rule as "an important driver of the shift toward community services" that are essential to mitigating the mental health crisis in this country. She called for the establishment of "an effective system of intensive community-based services, which have been shown to prevent or shorten hospitalizations."

Elsewhere in the world, good community care is beginning to supplement hospitalization. The most renowned example is in northern Italy, in the 220,000-person province of Trieste, where a community-based model is the exemplar lauded by the World Health Organization. A staff of 215 mental health workers operate four community mental health centers open twenty-four hours a day, seven days a week, for counseling, medication, home health care, housing, and other support services. Since Trieste's asylums were closed in 1978, this model has dramatically reduced suicides, hospitalizations, and mental health care costs. Today, there is but one "open" or unlocked psychiatric ward in town with a few beds, but staff there have found that inpatient care is rarely required.

Psychiatrist Robert Mezzina, MD, director of the Trieste program, has little use for classic mental hospitals. "Everywhere in the world when you have a psychiatric hospital—I've never seen a good one." Dr. Mezzina says care should instead be focused on "empowering people, human rights, and multisector intervention about housing, about work." His model is based on constant collaboration between patients and their families and mental health providers in the field, during home visits, and in their clinic. The focus is not on treating the diseases, he tells me, but on respecting and restoring the rights of the patient and coming up with reasonable solutions that are satisfactory to all parties. Thinking, as always, of Merle, I asked Dr. Mezzina, "What do you do when you cannot reason with a patient who is on a self-destructive path?"

Dr. Mezzina replied, "This happens only when we are too late, [when] the situation has gone too far."

Sure, but what then?

"Okay," he conceded, "we start to engage this person and try to gently, kindly offer some support and then try to engage the person—even in the streets—and then maybe offer what we call *hospitality* . . . the comfort of the community." The Trieste teams engage in "relentless negotiation" and try to talk the patient

into community-based treatment that includes meds and psychotherapy.

Can such an approach work in the United States, say, in a major
city? Unlike Los Angeles, the small town on the Mediterranean has
affordable housing, universal health insurance, and minimal drug
abuse problems. Still, Dr. Sherin thinks it's worth a shot. He and a
team of mental health and law enforcement officials have traveled
to Trieste to learn how to replicate their model. Meanwhile, Dr.
Mezzina has come to Los Angeles to share what he and his team
have learned. Despite the sociocultural differences between the two
locales, it is clear to me that we need to earnestly contemplate the
case of Trieste, which doesn't turn people with psychiatric disorders
into involuntary wards of the state. We also need social policy that
prevents sick people from self-destructing—dying, as Judy Harris
said, with their "civil liberties intact."

So far, the closest thing we have are the assertive community treatment (ACT) programs springing up across the country. The idea of
ACT, explains Dr. Swartz, is to provide the same wraparound services
that would be provided in a psychiatric hospital but within a home
setting. The service aims to be "a hospital without walls," where a
multidisciplinary team of nurses, social workers, and substance abuse
counselors provide in-home care with a ratio of about ten patients to
one staff member. "The ethos of that team," he explains, "is we will do
whatever it takes to help this person to live in the community. If they
need to go to the person's house every day and give them their medication, they will." As in Trieste, and just as Dr. Fenton did with Matthew Ornstein, the teams don't wait for a patient to come to them but
instead they meet ill individuals where they are. "They go see the patient at home and make sure they're getting what they need, taking
their medication, getting to whatever appointments they have,

learning how to live in the community. They'll take them shopping so that they know how to use their supermarkets—it's called *in vivo* rehabilitation." Today, many states have ACT programs for both court-mandated and voluntary patients, which have reduced both hospital-izations and jail time for participants.[12]

Another solution would be treatment facilities that people actu-ally want to be in. "Our system is so broken and so uninviting and unwelcoming and feels so unsafe that a lot of people don't want to engage in care," explains Dr. Sherin. "And because of that, they become gravely disabled. If our system were better and it embraced people and people felt okay, we wouldn't need involuntary treat-ment to this level."

Making treatment more inviting will require a cultural shift to-ward more respectful and welcoming care. It will mean providing decent housing and wraparound health care and avoiding chemical and physical restraints whenever possible. It may also mean a be-nevolent judge who requires that leveraged treatment program par-ticipants comply with some basic tenets like avoiding excessive drug and alcohol use, attending talk therapy sessions, seeking healthier lifestyle choices, and taking prescribed medications when they are essential to functioning. It will also require money. Not necessarily more money—as EDs and jails are very costly—but money that's better spent on addressing the underlying illnesses and the associ-ated social ills such as homelessness and poverty.

· · ·

Since the federal Affordable Care Act (ACA) took effect in 2010, many more adults have been covered for mental health care, particularly low-income individuals with insurance through the

Medicaid expansion.[13] The ACA also funded new programs for psychiatric care and incentivized the states to establish Health Homes, which provide coordinated case management for social services and medical and mental health care—a valuable approach for people at risk for multiple chronic disorders. The ACA has helped alleviate the discontinuities in coverage that made it difficult for people experiencing a first episode of psychosis to receive the services that research shows are critical to long-term outcomes.[14] It has also reduced the complications of being uninsured that result in delays in seeking help, reduced use of community treatment options, and increased likelihood of using only crisis or emergency services.[15]

"One of the more interesting features of the ACA," according to Dr. Goldman, "is that it makes coverage available to individuals before they become disabled and end up on SSI [Supplemental Security Income] or SSDI [Social Security Disability Insurance], which means that they have financial coverage to receive first-episode psychosis services—a new evidence-based suite of services. Prior to the ACA, most of the focus of the public sector was on individuals who were already disabled." In evaluating the role of ACA in the future of mental health care, we can't forget that a loss of protection for preexisting conditions—which often winds up on the political chopping block—would have disastrous results for people dependent on insurance from the health care exchange.

Another monumental piece of legislation is the Mental Health Parity and Addiction Equity Act, which took effect in 2010 yet continues to require monitoring and has spurred lawsuits against insurance companies that persist in discriminating against people with mental disorders. The law requires insurance companies to provide equal coverage for mental health as for general medical care.[16] Parity significantly reduces people's out-of-pocket expenses, explains Dr. Goldman. Today, "it's much harder to become bankrupted by a psychiatric health problem," which was easy to do before this federal legislation passed. The act also removed special limits on care for all mental disorders, including substance-related conditions, and numbers of outpatient visits or inpatient days. Instead, it offers coverage that better matches treatment protocols necessary in the real world. According to APA president Bruce Schwartz, MD, insurance companies "counted on [stigma] so that they could continue to discriminate against the care of the mentally ill, because no one was going to complain, or complain effectively."

Insurance carriers who've tried to skirt around parity and do business the old way are now getting schooled. In 2019, a federal judge ruled that the largest managed behavioral health care provider in the country, United Behavioral Healthcare, unlawfully denied mental health and substance abuse coverage to tens of thousands of adults and children.[17] The court found that although the insurance company did consistently cover urgent care (like acute and shorter hospitalizations for suicide attempts), they unlawfully denied coverage for stabilizing care (like residential and outpatient care to address the underlying illnesses).

One more sign that America is waking up to our mental health crisis is the 21st Century Cures Act of 2016, which launched additional research and treatment reforms. With bipartisan approval, the legislation also created a "mental health czar" position within the Department of Health and Human Services (HHS), now occupied by President Trump appointee Elinore McCance-Katz, MD, PhD. Previously, after two years as SAMHSA's first chief medical officer, she left after criticizing the agency for neglecting the treatment needs of "some of the most vulnerable in our society—those living with serious mental illness." She argued that "nowhere in SAMHSA's strategic initiatives is psychiatric treatment of mental illness a priority. . . . SAMHSA needs leadership that acknowledges the importance of addressing serious mental illness."[18]

In 2017, Dr. McCance-Katz returned to SAMHSA as the assistant secretary for mental health and substance use. One of her major goals, she tells me, is "making SAMHSA an agency that meets the needs of Americans living with serious mental illness. It's really very important that you use evidence-based practices, and that you work with American communities to make them aware of what evidence-based practices are."

Dr. McCance-Katz focuses on direct services, providing technical assistance, and giving out grants to fund community workshops, and she recently oversaw the launch of a clinical support system to provide national training to practitioners and organizations providing care. "It will focus on the kinds of enriched wraparound services that should, in our view, comprise assisted outpatient treatment. It will train on the medical aspects of the use of psychotropic medications, particularly second-generation antipsychotics, for which we have major medical concerns in the form of metabolic syndromes [i.e., obesity] that too often are not considered within the world of psychiatry, and because it's difficult for people with serious mental illness, often, to access physical health care."

Dr. McCance-Katz's understanding of the chronic medical conditions that often go hand in hand with SMI has led her to advocate strongly with HHS and with Congress for integrated physical and mental health care. With the benefit of additional funding, SAMHSA has been able to incorporate mental health care, SUD care, and physical health care into community-based programs, called Certified Community Behavioral Health Clinics (CCBHCs), that provide one-stop services. "This is very important because people with serious mental illness can have great difficulty navigating systems and have great need in all of those areas," Dr. McCance-Katz explains. These CCBHCs are also required to offer twenty-four-seven crisis intervention. "Too often, people languish in emergency departments with little care while they wait for a bed somewhere. They often never get that bed and will be released before they ever get any substantial service that they need for their illness," she says. "We think this will keep people out of EDs and help them to remain in communities where they can live very successfully with support." Other evidence-based services that SAMHSA recommends include first-episode psychosis programs and assertive community treatment, which she thinks of as "simply a first-episode-psychosis-type program, but for adults that have well-established and well-known psychotic disorders."

Dr. McCance-Katz's perspective is informed by her former position as medical director of a state hospital in Rhode Island. There she observed how many people came through the justice system after being charged with minor crimes. Had they received the services and treatment they needed, they likely could have avoided arrest. Just like Debbie, sitting in the women's prison in Los Angeles, many had been transferred for "competency restoration" and would be released with suboptimal follow-up; that is, they received the treatment they needed only while they were behind bars. "We shouldn't be doing that in the United States," says Dr. McCance-Katz. "That's not the way to treat serious mental illness." Her leadership on these issues has guided SAMHSA's efforts to provide training and technical assistance to criminal justice and diversion programs.

When I asked Dr. McCance-Katz what brought her to this work, she first gave me her curriculum vitae answer about her doctorate in infectious disease and epidemiology, followed by her shift to psychiatric research, and then to clinical pharmacology studies of the interactions between HIV medications and methadone. And then, for the first time in our lengthy conversation, there was silence. I waited for what came next. "I have had the opportunity to work with a lot of different types of folks and their families who've been affected by these disorders—substance use disorders, serious mental illnesses, medical illnesses. I had some family experience as well." She paused, careful to find the right words. "You know, we want to make things right for those we love. But we can't always do it. So, when you're a physician and you have the opportunity to work with others and maybe you can make a difference in their lives. It's been my privilege to be able to do that. I don't want to say much more than that." I had no intention of pressing her further. While I can't presume anything about the specific family circumstances that drive her work, it does give me hope to think that someone who has significant power to determine how our nation addresses serious mental illness may be yet another member of the tribe.

Since 2010, we've seen some real advances. Still, getting good mental health care is very difficult. Even if you have the best health care coverage in the world, many mental health professionals don't accept insurance because of the onerous paperwork and relatively low reimbursement rates. People lucky enough to have out-of-network coverage can see providers by paying them out of pocket and waiting for reimbursement—but even these plans often also have huge deductibles that require extraordinary up-front expenditures. For most people, the cost of care continues to present a significant barrier to getting and maintaining mental health. Although the ACA and parity made critical advancements to our fractured system, mental health advocates say that truly quality psychiatric care will emerge only with the establishment of a universal, single-payer insurance system of the sort used in every other industrialized country in the world. In a 2018 paper published in the *International Journal of Health Services*, political scientist David A. Rochefort emphasized that the ACA is just a start. Although it has been correctly lauded as revolutionary, "tens of millions of Americans still lack health insurance, insurance companies are resisting the implementation of parity coverage rule, and inequalities in the financing and organization of care continue to worsen in key respects."[19]

Universal health care creates incentives for people to stay healthy, says Dr. Miranda. "In a system like that, where everyone is in it and we're all paying for each other's health care, the system itself is highly motivated to keep people healthy. If you can catch people [early] and give them good care, it's much cheaper than having them end up in jails, and in and out of ERs, and in and out of psychiatric hospitalization."

• • •

Many advocates see the mental health crisis as giving rise to a new civil rights movement. "If this were cancer, there'd be a revolution in this country," says Patrick Kennedy, in his keynote at the 2016 annual national meeting of NAMI. Since retiring from Congress in 2011 to focus on his own recovery from substance abuse and bipolar disorder, he has founded the Kennedy Forum, a nonprofit aimed at transforming mental health and addiction care delivery. "This is . . . a civil rights issue. It's about the discrimination against our brothers and sisters simply because of the immutable fact [that] their illness is an illness of the brain as opposed to an illness of any other organ in the body."

Like the civil rights movement on behalf of people of color, a mental health civil rights movement of advocates and people with SMI determined to fight for fair treatment is pushing us forward into a new era. These two movements are intersecting as well. David Satcher, MD, is the sixteenth surgeon general of the United States and founder of the Satcher Health Leadership Institute at the Morehouse School of Medicine. I asked Dr. Satcher, a black freedom fighter who marched with Dr. Martin Luther King Jr., how his fight today for folks with mental illness compares to his fight for civil rights in the 1960s. Without hesitation, Dr. Satcher tells me that this mental illness battle is "harder by far." He goes on to remind me about the responsibility we all have to take a stand, explaining that he takes particular inspiration from Rosa Parks, the black woman whose arrest for refusing to sit at the back of a bus launched the Montgomery bus boycott in 1955. "Years later, she was back in Detroit where she grew up and they asked her, 'What was it like? How did you arrive at this decision that you were willing to go to jail to keep your seat, when you'd been giving it up all these years?' And she just said, 'I just made up my mind.' She said, 'You know, I don't think there's anything more powerful than a made-up mind.'"

Patrisse Khan-Cullors definitely has *a made-up mind*. In 2014, she was spending mornings in front of the county jail, handing out flyers to anyone who would take them, to fight against incarceration. In 2015, with a bullhorn and a snare drum accompanist, she led a group of twenty or so demonstrators protesting Los Angeles's plan to "throw away the mentally ill" with chants of "No justice, no peace." "We may be small," she said to the folks holding home-made signs who'd assembled outside Twin Towers, "but we are a mighty force."

Three years later, as we crawl through the five thirty a.m. rush-hour traffic of Los Angeles on September 26, 2017, she tells me the slogan for today's planned protest: "You can't get well in a cell." A few hours later, Patrisse would lead that chant among the nearly one hundred protesters who've come to speak out against the con-struction of a new mental health jail in Los Angeles. Her plan is to block the street with one hundred jail beds that she and a team of fellow artists built as a visual symbol of the additional treatment—rather than incarceration—beds that Los Angeles County needs. "We have historically *not* fought for people with mental illness and severe mental illness," she says. "We've chosen as a culture, as a country, as people, to lock them up in hospitals and now prison facilities."

That morning, she and her collaborators drive a caravan of five U-Haul trucks into the middle of downtown's Temple Street. A team of young-adult volunteers, a multicultural group of different races, ages, and genders, unload the handmade cots in front of the County Board of Supervisors building, blocking traffic. The pro-testers flood the street while the group's lawyer interfaces with the police to prevent the authorities from thwarting the unloading of the beds. No one gets hurt. No one is arrested. But like the civil rights activists of the 1960s, these volunteers are prepared to go to jail for a cause greater than themselves.

"This, for us, is about life or death. This place, this city, this county, has deeply neglected the people that I love, and I'm tired of it," Patrisse says. "I'm tired of them getting away with whatever they want to get away with and not considering the impact it has on real human lives." And "if we can stop the mental health jail, I think we will have put forward a new trend, hopefully, across the nation. We have to be a part of a growing movement that's saying folks with mental health issues deserve to have a life that's not just about survival but that's about thriving. Part of protesting and showing up and getting in elected officials' faces is trying to change the course of history." Patrisse's demonstration today is aimed not only at lifting up people with SMI but also at reducing the epidemic of incarceration that has wreaked destruction across the nation.

When I met Monte, I asked to meet his sister for no other reason than to ask her permission to follow Monte and his family. I had no idea that she was an activist. No idea that over the next few years, she would become one of the most vocal and recognized civil rights activists of the twenty-first century. I never imagined that she would end up taking me to my first mental health protest—or that it would become perhaps the most important such protest of the century. I never imagined that she (and all the people I've followed as part of this project) would help me overcome my own shame and silence.

CHAPTER 9

GOING HOME

The last time I saw Merle was on her fifty-fifth birthday. I'd taken the train to Philadelphia for one more ill-fated attempt to convince my sister to move someplace cleaner and safer. With my hand on the familiar wrought-iron railing of my childhood home, I climbed the stairs under the beige steel awning with scalloped trim that was identical to all the other awnings over the doors of all the other semidetached row houses on the block. Merle peeked out the still-chained front door.

"They're here, aren't they?"

No, they weren't. No, I hadn't called the police. Nevertheless, Merle wasn't taking any chances. She refused to open the door. I sat on the stoop, hoping she might change her mind. I wondered if I should force my way in but knew that would only lead to a confrontation even worse than those we'd had before my mom died. I didn't want any more scenes.

The convalescent home I'd found was prepared to accept her, and on the phone, Merle kept saying she was nearly ready to go. "Next week," "next month," she told me throughout the fall. But some combination of her disease and her traumatic memories of being dragged to hospitals had left her afraid of doctors; she kept stalling to avoid the required medical examination. I wanted to keep my promise to my mother. I wanted to finally realize my lifelong goal to help my sister get well.

A month later, in November, I called and told her, "You *will* move out. Not forever. Just long enough to get help. Long enough to get the house back into some livable condition." *And maybe*, I thought, *long enough for me to get legal custody and have a judge rule that she has to accept treatment.*

I wasn't backing down this time. My mother was no longer around to yell at me. "I'll make you."

"You'll never get away with it," she screamed.

The arguments over the telephone continued into December— until she stopped picking up. For two weeks, many times each day, I would call, but no one ever answered. I had called Family Services in Philadelphia a month earlier, but it would take weeks for them to send an assessment team. I didn't press them; Merle wouldn't let them in anyway. Even if she did, who knew what they would find inside or how she would react. I worried that their arrival could precipitate a visit by the police. My parents' lawyer advised me against involving the city officials in any way. He said that if Merle entered the "system" they might take over her life and seize the house. With no good options, I waited some more. But now, Merle wasn't answering.

I finally dialed my brother-in-law Bob, Gail's widower, who was the closest relative living in the area. Bob and I had always had an easy relationship. I thought of him as my smart, well-bred older brother. Over the decades of his marriage to my sister, I had come to value his perspective as someone who was close to us but had sufficient distance to maintain a useful clearsightedness that neither Gail nor I possessed. Bob had been an executive in the food business but in retirement, he had trained for his certification as a licensed social worker and provided psychotherapy at a local community mental health clinic. I had no doubt that he was the right person to call, and I was grateful to have him in my corner. I asked him to go to my sister's house.

Bob called. He said he knocked on the front door, over and over; then he tried the back door. I knew what I had to do, despite every order issued by parents and relatives over a lifetime. Then I asked him to wait until the squad car arrived.

"The police need to break down the door," he said when he called me back a short time later.

"Tell them to go in through the back door, the basement door," I advised. "It's the easiest one." Then I held the line, looking at the emptied dinner plates while my family went about their evening routines. Across from me, my wife sat at her laptop preparing a lecture for her college English class, my daughter was doing homework upstairs, and my son and his girlfriend listened to music in his room.

As I waited, my head swam with memories. Merle had been my first playmate. She would curl up on the floor with me and our dog to watch television. She was the same sister who, just two months earlier, had locked me out of the house when I came from New York to celebrate our birthdays, which were only a few days apart. I thought about how as soon as I got my license at sixteen—the same age my son was now—I had dropped her off at the hospital and watched her get yanked in by the aides, the slam of the metal door echoing as she yelled back at me. I remembered the "best" hospitalization at the private Friends Hospital, where she'd received electroshock therapy. I recalled holding Merle's hand in the limo after burying our mother. Just the two us in the car, we were the last remaining members of our family. As we passed the grave-stones, she smiled and said cheerfully, as though speaking to someone else, "I have the most wonderful brother. He will always take care of me." "Of course," I replied. It was the closest I'd felt to her, and the most hopeful I'd felt about her future, in years.

"Merle is dead," Bob said. "They found her in your parents' bed." He waited as the police investigated the scene and the coroner certified her death, but never entered the house. "I guess I didn't want to see her lying in the bed dead," he later told me.

The autopsy cited a heart attack as the immediate cause of death, with a breast cancer lesion, long undiagnosed and untreated, as secondary. But I knew the truth: what killed my sister was serious mental illness, complete with its accompanying shame, stubbornness, denial, and confusion.

I arranged a funeral. I gave one more eulogy, this time to just a few cousins, and buried the last member of my family of origin.

Left with the responsibility of cleaning out my childhood home, I decided to let it all go. What was I going to do with an out-of-tune, broken-down piano 120 miles from my home? Memories of delighting my mother and sisters with my attempts at honky-tonk weren't enough to save it. I didn't need the huge dining room table or the matching mahogany breakfront, still filled with dishes and silverware; it had been forty years since I'd turned on its display lights to show company what a fine home we had. Who needed the secretary that shelved the World Books or the books themselves, which I'd read over and over, cover to cover? The crystal chandelier, the wooden panels depicting medieval minstrels, the statuettes of the Venus de Milo. I wanted to put everything behind me. I hung on to the small metal menorah; the glass dish, stained brownish along the edges, in a metal cradle that kept the Rosh Hashanah brisket warm; and, of course, the family photo albums. When I was eight years old, I started my career as a documentarian. I decided to be the keeper of our beautiful family's photo history. My parents stored the albums that I made in the bottom drawers of the secretary, along with important documents such as birth certificates. The photo books came out on holidays. They were the lifeblood of our family: who we were, or who we thought we were. How we wanted to be remembered.

On the first page of the first album, all five of us pose in the old house in a working-class neighborhood in Philadelphia. My parents sit side by side on the couch with infant me between them, my father's large hands—the hands of a former amateur prizefighter—supporting his only son. He's in a tweed suit and a striped dress shirt buttoned all the way to the top, and he wears the gold Art Deco watch that I would ultimately call my own. Beside him is my mother, a redhead whose smile and elegance, I still believe, rivaled Rita Hayworth's. There in polka dots is my tall, slightly awkward sister Gail at age twelve. She smiles broadly, her hands on my father's shoulders. Next to my mother, in an organdy dress and petticoat with puff sleeves and lace ruffles, my six-year-old sister Merle beams, confident and relaxed. It's the least constricted and most self-possessed I've ever seen her.

I shipped those few things to New York. Then I was done.

• • •

When I began this project in 2012, I hadn't set out to speak about my family even though my need to tell this story was set in motion in response to my personal experience. In fact, I am professionally trained in the art of avoiding self-disclosure. As a young psychiatrist, I was taught to remain circumspect about what I tell patients about my own life, views, and responses. My job is to understand and help my patients, not burden them with my own baggage. Yet I've come to realize that as a filmmaker, a writer, and now, unexpectedly, an activist, my obligation is to speak the entire truth. To hide behind a shield of detached professionalism is just another excuse to hide behind the veil of shame and secrecy. How could I continue to hide when I had spent the past seven years convincing Monte, Patrisse, Johanna, Delilah, Todd, Debbie, and Dr. McGhee to share their stories? To understand my story, I needed to go back home.

The first weekend of October 2017, the week of my sixtieth birthday, and what would have been Merle's sixty-sixth, I take the train to Thirtieth Street Station, the stop where I always disembarked on what were, for a time, regular visits home. Bob picks me up and we drive a few miles to the grounds of what was once the Pennsylvania Hospital. Gone is the institution for people with schizophrenia, bipolar disorder, and other SMIs. Now, the old institute is divided into two parts: a beautiful rehabilitation center for substance abuse and a dilapidated homeless shelter used by the city to house families in crisis.

Turning off Market Street, we pull into the same driveway that I last saw forty-seven years earlier, during Merle's first hospitalization. I am by no means the first person to journey up this pathway with no idea of what lies ahead. Back in 1752, Benjamin Franklin had cofounded the original Pennsylvania Hospital in Center City. Then, from 1836 to 1841, the stately buildings of the Pennsylvania Hospital for the Insane were constructed on 101 acres of farmland in North Philadelphia.[1] When the facility opened, one hundred mental patients from the original Center City hospital were brought by carriages to the new asylum. From that day forward, people with psychiatric disorders traversed this same terrain, from the days of horse-drawn paddy wagons until the days of police vans like the one that brought Merle here in 1971. Families like mine followed until, in 1997—in an era of declining insurance payments, when treating serious mental illness simply didn't pay—the nation's first mental hospital, Merle's first mental hospital, closed.

With permission from the rehab center's management, Bob and I venture inside and find a room not unlike the one I'd sat in with my family at age fourteen, where the psychiatrist's bike had hung on the wall amid shelves filled with books. We sit down in the refurbished conference room with high ceilings and white painted moldings at a long table ringed with half a dozen red leather chairs. Bob tells me how relieved he and Gail had felt when they'd arrived here with Merle in the police van. The psychiatrist they'd met with quickly took charge, explaining that they'd give Merle an injection to calm her down. Bob felt she was in good hands. "We thought we were doing the right thing up until your father called me," he recalls. "He called me on the phone, he was so angry. He had never been so angry at me before that time. He was yelling at me on the phone. I was at work."

Bob tried to reason with him. "I said, 'Well, it's just like if someone cuts themselves badly, you have to take them to the hospital. She needed the help.'"

"*Never* do that again," Bob says, channeling my father. "You never, never do that ever again. Never. It's my daughter and you're not to do anything like that ever again."

"Do you think he just didn't want the situation to be out of his control?" I ask.

"I think with him, it was shame. I think there was a lot of shame regarding mental illness with him." I learn that Bob and Gail had continued for years to urge my parents to get more care for Merle, but they wouldn't hear of it.

I tell Bob about the few fraught family therapy sessions we'd had before my father pulled Merle out. I tell him about how I'd looked up to the psychiatrist and how I'd forged a solidarity with Gail— both of us allied around the idea that Merle was sick and needed help despite my parents' denial.

Bob and I leave the rehab center and walk through the less maintained buildings that today serve homeless families. As Philadelphia's largest nonprofit homeless shelter, the building provides emergency housing in sixty-five individual rooms and has case managers to help with health, education, and long-term housing needs. All across the nation, the sites of former asylums have been turned over to homeless shelters and jails. Dr. Torrey often mentions how the North Carolina mental hospital that reformer Dorothea Dix had founded in 1856 closed in October 2016 and was replaced by a jail on the very same plot of land.

As Bob and I drive through the city, I am reminded of all the good things about Philadelphia: the Parkway where Rocky ran up the stairs of the art museum, the diverse population, Pat's cheesesteaks, and the trendy restaurants downtown. Still, ghosts appear. As we pass through Rittenhouse Square I remember driving the same route as a teenager, seeing a bag lady on the sidewalk, and realizing that bag lady was in fact my sister, roaming the streets in the throes of psychosis.

After lunch, Bob and I turn down my old street. When I was five, we'd moved here from a poor part of North Philly like the Beverly Hillbillies arriving at their mansion. My first glimpse of the long row of brick homes, each with its own driveway and little piece of lawn, felt like heaven on earth; and for a time, it was. It looks as homey to me now as it did when we pulled up the first time.

As we approach the house, Bob whispers, "It's weird because I have so many memories with coming here. A lot of events, you know? Holidays, and dinners, and just so many things. And some unhappy things. You know? Pretty unhappy things."

I have my memories, too. On summer Sundays, kids in the neighborhood darted through sprinklers and splashed in inflatable kiddie pools while adults lounged on postage-stamp porches or fixed their cars. One Sunday when I was eleven and Merle was seventeen, Dad was under the hood of his red 1967 Pontiac Firebird convertible, shirt off, soaking up the sun, tinkering. "Al, you're always playing with your cars!" my mom would often jokingly complain, wanting more of his attention. But on this day, what she wanted from him was intervention.

From where I lay in a notch between the bushes in the front yard, sunbathing with one of those folding reflectors that were popular at the time, I could hear Merle ratcheting up, her high-pitched voice anxious, twisting, angling for a fight. My mother screamed back. Merle was asking for something and refusing to accept no for an answer. I tried not to listen. Then the hitting started. "Al! Al! Where are you?!?" my mother hollered. "Al, do you hear what's going on here?"

Dad emerged from under the hood, engine still running, dropped his tools, swung open the screen door, and stormed through the house. Suddenly Merle burst through the door and ran down the front walk. I watched as she climbed into the driver's seat. She drove down the street with the hood still up.

Whenever my sister was calm, the musical score in my head was Bobby Hebb's song "Sunny." But when she lost control, I heard Cream's live version of "Crossroads," with Eric Clapton's frenetic guitar screaming over the pounding drums and bass. As the tires of Dad's beloved convertible bumped off the curb, Clapton's guitar licks screeched through my head. Children spraying each other with hoses stopped short. Sunbathing moms raised their sunglasses. The whole neighborhood gawked at the spectacle of the Rosenberg family's red Firebird swerving down the street. Our insanity had finally bled beyond the walls of our house. I felt like Roy Scheider's character in *Jaws*, when he realizes the shark will attack his son and the camera dolly zooms in just as his world collapses with the understanding of the terror that is about to unfold. For me, the terror was having my worst secret broadcast to everyone on my block.

A new family, immigrants from Eastern Europe, live here now. They've turned it into a warm home, decorated in bright reds and yellows, the walls hung with family portraits. They welcome us in and sit us down on the living room sofa. "Must bring back lots of memories," says the family's twenty-something daughter as her grandmother serves cookies and juice on a platter. "Brings back memories," I answer. "Can I look around?"

In the living room, I lose my breath. It's as if this family has found our old dining room table and breakfront and filled it with their own dishes and religious ornaments. In the dining room, I can still see us all gathered around the table for Jewish holidays, replete with toasts and blessings, my parents never happier, the welcoming sunshine of Gail's smile, grandchildren gathered around the piano. Then, Merle making an appearance. On one of these holidays, I'd had my video camera fixed on her as she came downstairs, hands on the railing. "How are you?" she asked me. My mother exclaimed, "Oh, my. Wonderful!" I can still feel her tremendous hope that Merle's long-awaited arrival at the dinner table meant that she was well, and we were whole once again.

Now, almost three decades later, hands on the same wooden banister finished with a gold ornament on top, Bob and I walk up the carpeted stairs. Around the corner in the upstairs hall, the bathroom looks like I remembered. This is where almost all of Merle's fights had ended.

We enter the room that had been my parents', and I flash back to the night in 2003 when Merle's hoarding had overflowed from her bedroom and taken over the house. She had stacked the bed high with clothing. Crowded out of her own room, my sick mother, then in her late eighties, wound up sleeping on the sofa, during what ended up being her last days at home. When Merle refused to move her stuff, I had had enough. Just like my father, I was determined to fix it all by force. I grabbed the clothes so that my mother could lie down, and Merle erupted into a long tirade that ended with a howl. "Now you did it!" she screamed. Merle cursed me as I threw her clothes on the ground. "Now, you did it! The curse will continue with you!" she shouted, threatening that her demons would strike me next.

My mother reprimanded me, too. "You come from New York to make trouble!"

A few days later, my mother was hospitalized for dehydration. She died in the hospital.

Bob and I enter Merle's room. Its walls have been painted a soothing blue-gray, the bed neatly topped with a geometric-patterned quilt. The screen in the window above the driveway is broken, the torn triangular corner dangling outside the glass. I look down at the smooth slope of the driveway three stories below, where I made my escape to Boston, forty years earlier.

I tell Bob, "I don't really know how to make sense of it all, honestly."

"There may be things you can never figure out, you know?" he replies gently.

I think back on all the patients I've spoken with over the years—family members torn apart by their loved ones' illnesses, all those who faced the impossible task of stopping their loved ones' unstoppable self-destruction, forced to fight with people who thwarted all their attempts at sanity and order.

In 2019, in the *New York Times Magazine* advice column The Ethicist, a mother asked if she could cut her daughter out of her life.[2] "I am the parent of a high school student with multiple issues," she wrote. "Her learning disabilities are dwarfed by a severe mood disorder. Nearly two decades of this severe mood has forced our family to endure daily, hour-long tantrums." She listed a familiar litany of problems with neighbors and police, medication refusal, and the bedlam that had "battered our marriage and careers." She described having "lost the middle chunk of my life to chaos and misery." She asked The Ethicist, Kwame Anthony Appiah, "Am I condemned to live this way until I die?" Appiah responded, "Our culture demonizes parental ambivalence," and advised the mother to seek psychiatric consultation.

I can't fault Appiah's response, but I know that even as a psychiatrist, I struggle to find answers. The best I can muster is what I tell Bob that day in my sister's bedroom: "I know what my mother must have felt. I just cannot find words to make sense out of it, except to say it was a horrible illness, horrible for my mother. It was horrible for my father. It was horrible for everyone, and mostly it was horrible for Merle. I just wish there were a happier ending to her life, and to my entire family's life."

Before returning to New York, I have one more stop to make—one more place I've never wanted to visit: the cemetery where the bodies of my parents and Merle now rest.

I hate anything having to do with death. For as long as I can remember I had worried about being twelve years younger than Gail. It scared me that one day I'd be visiting my family in a place like this. All my life, I'd avoided even looking at graveyards. As a kid, I'd crouch in the back of the car behind the front seat whenever we'd pass a cemetery to avoid looking at it. But Bob knows cemeteries. After Gail's death, Bob regularly visited the plot they'd purchased twenty miles away. He kept a steady supply of small rocks in his car from trips to Martha's Vineyard where he and Gail had spent their summers.

When we arrive, Bob brings me to my parents' grave first. Dad died in 1992. Buried next to him was my mother, who died in 2003. "Goes by fast," Bob says, handing me a small rock to place on their headstones.

"Goes by fast," I echo.

Then with the roar of the state highway behind us, he leads me to Merle's grave a few yards away in a section empty of any other headstones. "She's all alone," I observe.

Her monument is inscribed with the words I'd written: "Devoted and beloved daughter, sister, cousin, aunt, friend. Forever in our hearts and minds." I place a Martha's Vineyard pebble on the smooth top edge.

"Aren't we supposed to say a prayer?"

"The Kaddish," Bob replies.

"Do you know the Kaddish?"

"I don't know it by heart, no."

"Do you know part of it?"

"*Yitgadal v'yitkadash sh'mei raba b'alma di-v'ra . . .*" he begins. "It goes on and on. . . ."

"Do you know what it means?"

"It's just about saying you still believe in God even though, you know, bad things happen." This marks the end of our day together. The sun is setting, and the orange rays highlight the grass and soil as the wind dies down.

I turn to Bob. "It's really not bad here."

"No, the sun's coming right in over here. It shines right on your family's grave right at this time of day. On a good day, it shines right on the graves."

"Really? A *good* day is when the sun shines on the graves?"

With his hand on my shoulder, walking to the car, I felt the familiar warmth of family.

• • •

On my way back to Manhattan, I recall something Johanna said, with tears in her eyes, during our last interview. "When I first got sick, I remember how scared and alone I felt. It would have been nice to know that there are others like this." She took a deep breath. "So, if you have this," she said, addressing her message to anyone who might need it, "you're not alone."

We are not alone. But we desperately need one another. We need to share our stories. We need comradery and a unified movement. As many of us have found out the hard way, none of us can fix these diseases alone. None of us, rich or poor, can insulate and protect our family members from psychiatric disorders. I've met billionaires who are helpless to get their ill children out of jail. I've met the most powerful public health officials who have helplessly watched their siblings die on the streets. The richest among us can't buy medicines that don't exist; the cleverest person can't find a bed in a hospital that lies in ruins; the smartest doctor can't unravel the riddle of these poorly understood brain diseases. We can only solve this together, as an outspoken, unified, undeterred, and unashamed community.

The strength of that sort of community was on full display on

February 12, 2019, when Patrisse Khan-Cullors and other activists including Dr. Dias protested at the Los Angeles County Board of Supervisors' meeting under the banner of their group, JusticeLA-Now. Dr. Dias spoke out based on his twelve years in the trenches as LAC+USC's director of psychiatry. He had dealt day in and day out with the mental health crisis overwhelming the hospital until he finally quit in 2017 out of concern that the stress was bad for his *own* health. (Dr. McGhee had also quit, one year earlier.)

On this landmark February day, Dr. Dias added his voice to the voices of dozens of other psychiatrists who attended the meeting of the County Board of Supervisors to demand that they halt plans to build the new mental health jail. To me, this jail had always seemed a foregone conclusion. When the project was approved by the Los Angeles Board of Supervisors in June 2018, it seemed like Patrisse's hundred-bed protest in 2017 had been too little, too late. But she and other activists refused to give up. When the JusticeLANow coalition arrived at the meeting, they listened as none other than Los Angeles Department of Mental Health director Dr. Jonathan Sherin, Department of Health director Dr. Christina Ghaly, and Community Mental Health director Dr. Mark Ghaly spoke out against the planned facility. They heard Dr. Mark Ghaly say, "You can't get well in a cell."

That day history was made. Above a photo showing Patrisse among her crew of protesters, the *Los Angeles Times* headline read: "In Landmark Move, LA County Will Replace Men's Central Jail with a Mental Health Hospital for Inmates."[3] *They did it.* The supervisors reversed their decision to build a 3,800-bed mental health jail in the spot where Men's Central Jail now stands—the same spot where Patrisse had stood with a handful of ragtag demonstrators four years earlier.

This reversal was an inspiring piece of activism that happened because people joined forces to fight for viable and humane solutions. "I can't stop crying," Patrisse texted me hours after the vote. Without a doubt their tireless efforts had prevented innumerable tears that would have been shed by incarcerated people and their loved ones had the mental "health" jail been erected.

After the protest, I dreamed I was working in a small psychiatric emergency department, similar to the LAC+USC psych ED, only smaller. I was in the admissions and triage area, with a calm and dutiful doctor and nurse. No fighting and no restraints. It was like any small quiet ED, but for the fact that this ED was (somehow) an annex of Philadelphia's 30th Street Station. I was called to the information desk in the heart of the train station. Merle was there with her suitcase, waiting. Standing tall, showered, and best of all, happy to see me, she was eager to be admitted, to get well. We smiled at each other. Then, as she took my hand, we walked toward the annexed hospital. No contests of wills. No yelling. No cursing. No battles. And, still in my dream, I thought to myself, "I finally found it: a happy ending!" Then I woke up and realized all over again that Merle was gone.

While there is no Hollywood ending for me and Merle, something unprecedented is happening now in America. We are no longer standing by helplessly as our family members get thrown away by society, without care, taking outdated medicines, living in cells or on the streets. We are no longer cowering in the corners. We are no longer silent. I am no longer alone.

PRACTICAL ADVICE FOR PERSONS WITH SMI AND THEIR FAMILIES

While activists push for care and cures, researchers advance the science, and politicians and thought leaders promote societal and policy change, today's patients, health care providers, concerned citizens, and family members need immediate, practical answers. If a doctor diagnoses you with strep throat, the remedy—an antibiotic—is obvious, inexpensive, and easy to procure. When it comes to mental illness, solutions are not so clear-cut. The recommendations that follow are a compilation of the best I've heard from experts, mental health care consumers, and families. For more suggestions, please go to the websites and books of experts like Lloyd Sederer, MD, Xavier Amadour, PhD, and DJ Jaffe.

1. **Connect with NAMI.** For solidarity, education, advice, and to find knowledgeable service providers, call the National Alliance on Mental Illness, the nation's largest grassroots mental health organization. The HelpLine (800-950-6264), operated by NAMI staff and volunteers, and their website provide information and resources, including the following:

- Symptoms of mental health conditions
- Treatment options
- Local support groups and services
- Educational programs
- Helping family members get treatment
- Employment programs
- Legal issues, including listings of attorneys with expertise and experience representing people living with mental health conditions

In addition to information and resources, NAMI provides opportunities for connecting with others coping with similar challenges. This solidarity can help us find the strength to shake off the stigma of mental illness and recognize it as a health condition that deserves the same respect, attention, and support, societal and otherwise, as any other. Support and advocacy groups for families can offer a stable base that fuels the resilience necessary to fight for the policy change that is so urgently needed in our time.

The burden on parents whose young or adult children develop SED or SMI is tremendous. The attempts they make to get them to go to school, get a job, see a therapist, or take medicine can wind up in fights that lead to violence or even suicide. If a parent decides not to push, their child may draw inward or self-medicate with street drugs. People blame these families for "enabling"— for having no backbone and setting no limits—but it is incumbent on the rest of us to quit the blame game and instead make sure that families have the resources and wherewithal to find proper treatment. NAMI is a great first step to helping families deal with self-doubt, blame, and second-guessing, and to find viable solutions.

Other excellent resources are available at Strong365 (https://strong365.org/), an empowering online community and resource hub for young people and their families seeking information and support for early stage psychosis.

2. **Develop a crisis plan.** Coping with SMI is like living in a city that's under constant threat of terrorist attack. You need to plan for the worst. The first step is to research what resources are available in your community. Call the nearest psychiatric emergency room to see if they have a mobile crisis unit. These teams usually include mental health professionals who can perform a home visit for the purpose of evaluation, provide referrals to outpatient treatment, and, if necessary, hospitalize someone in immediate danger to self or others. The social worker, nurse, or doctor will be able to tell you what the mobile crisis team can provide and how to contact them. Now, before disaster hits, is the perfect time to write this number down on your emergency list.

3. **Create a support team.** Monte and his family provide an excellent model of how to build a support team around a loved one with SMI. Patrisse has learned how to manage what she can but also how to involve others, helping them to step into various roles: the person to take Monte to the hospital, the one to bring him food, and the friendly faces to rescue him when his

psychosis escalates. Like me, Patrisse has found that sometimes as a sibling, you are too close to be helpful, too angry to engage, or simply too busy. It's important to marshal outside resources for everyone's well-being.

In 1980, the average hospital stay for someone with schizophrenia was forty-two days.[1] Today it is seven days or less, and often just three to four days.[2] Since aftercare is usually lacking, loved ones wind up filling in the gaps. Family members would do well to avail themselves of all the support they can get from friends and relatives. We know that what works best for people with SMI are unified teams of professionals where social workers, psychologists, psychiatrists, and vocational and housing specialists all work together under a team leader toward a unified cause of support. When outside resources like that aren't available, loved ones banding together can keep the burden from falling on any one or two individuals.

4. **Prioritize empathy and collaboration.** People with SMI can quickly become marginalized and alienated from their own treatment. Collaboration is critical not only to preserving relationships but also to maintaining the human connection that is an essential element of healing. Striving for allegiance can go a long way toward fostering a team approach.

I don't want to minimize the difficulty of collaborating with someone with a brain disorder. Many people wind up living in an altered form of reality, and it can be difficult to find common ground. One thing I can say with certainty is that issuing "my way or the highway" ultimatums often backfires. Addiction specialists often encourage families to take a "tough love" approach that can include withdrawing financial support if the loved one won't accept medical help. That message may be able to break through to people who are addicted to substances, but for someone who is experiencing a psychotic episode—who doesn't ever "sober up" but instead remains "intoxicated" with their delusions, hallucinations, and irritable moods—this advice does not apply. My sister would sooner perish than accept medical intervention. That's why most experts put at the top of their advice list to never deny health insurance, medical care, shelter, or food. What *does* help is offering up as much love as you can.

Norm Ornstein learned this painful lesson with Matthew. "For years I would try to reason and argue with Matthew based on my powers of logic," he tells me, "but it was very clear that there was nothing that I was going to say that would shake him from his own beliefs." Following his failed attempts to reason his son into treatment, it became clear that he needed to find a different approach. Dr. Xavier Amador's seminal book *I Am Not Sick: I Don't Need Help* offers a new model for communication: the Listen-Empathize-Agree-Partner (LEAP) method, which emphasizes the human connection above all else.

The core tools of LEAP, which is specifically geared toward gently nudging someone with SMI to accept treatment, are "Listening (using 'reflective' listening), Empathizing (strategically—especially about those feelings you've ignored during your previous arguments about your loved one being sick and needing treatment), Agreeing (on those things you can agree on and agreeing to disagree about the others), and ultimately Partnering (forming a partnership to achieve the goals you share)."[3] This approach hinges on finding connection points, which fosters mutual respect.

What if a loved one refuses treatment because they are convinced they aren't sick? The phenomenon, called anosognosia, or poor insight, is a symptom of the disordered thinking caused by the disease itself. It's important to keep in mind that this lack of recognition is not a choice, but a part of the sickness.

You don't have to agree with your loved one's reality, Amador insists, "but you *do* need to listen and *genuinely* respect it." Reflective listening, whereby you take in what the other person is saying with an open mind, without being reactive, and then restate what you've heard in order to "reflect" it back, is key. It sets the stage for the next steps of empathizing, agreeing, and partnering toward your shared goals. The first objective is to repair any damage to the relationship from your previous attempts at rational convincing. The second is to help the ill individual find their own motivations for accepting treatment by presenting medication or therapy as a means for them to fulfill their own wishes.[4] This protocol not only makes common sense, it's rooted in long-standing clinical practices that have been used successfully for generations. It remains one of our best defenses against engaging in a one-on-one power play in which all parties lose.

5. **Get psychiatric help.** If at all possible, it's best to think through your options before a crisis arises. (See

number 2.) But when trouble starts, trust your instincts and get help sooner rather than later. The resources available will depend on your location, but Dr. Amador recommends the following:

If an emergency room visit is needed, accompany your loved one. When dealing with hospitals and/or mental health providers who refuse to speak to you as a friend or family member, consider taking Norm's advice not to let them use an overly wide interpretation of HIPAA (the Health Insurance Portability and Accountability Act). In his experience, "almost everybody tries to hide behind HIPAA to avoid the hassles or the potential lawsuits." For many health care providers, particularly overburdened staff in the hospital, it often is more convenient to invoke privacy rules than to put effort into parsing out what information they might be able to share with families (which doctors may fear could risk backlash in the form of a lawsuit for privacy infraction or even evoking the patient's anger). Norm urges family members to request a copy of the institution's medical information privacy policy, read it, and point out any discrepancies between what is written and their blanket refusal to provide any information at all.

Ron Honberg, a lawyer with NAMI, explains that medical information can be shared with loved ones when the "health provider determines, based on professional judgment, that doing so is in the best interests of his/her patient" or "believes, based on professional judgment, that patient does not have capacity to agree or object, and sharing information is in his/her best interests."

The Treatment Advocacy Center also points out that

"providers are not precluded under HIPAA from *accepting* information from families or others who are knowledgeable about the individual and his or her treatment needs. [In other words, there is no law against the doctor hearing a family member's concerns, history, or experiences with the ill individual.] A good medical provider will want to know all the relevant information available. If your loved one's provider refuses to listen to your information, contact a supervisor such as the hospital administrator, insist that you be heard, and/or submit written information."

If you need emergency intervention at home, call the local crisis intervention team (CIT). To find out if one is in your community, call any psychiatric emergency room or your local police department. Members of these teams, which often include some combination of a doctor, nurse, social worker, and case manager, are trained to deal with people in mental health crises and therefore better equipped to interpret behavior as a symptom of SMI rather than of criminal intent.

As Dr. Amador explains, if a mobile crisis team judges "that hospitalization is warranted, they will try to convince your loved one to accompany them to the hospital. If he refuses, they can initiate the commitment process immediately."[5]

Assertive community treatment programs are another resource. Lloyd Sederer, MD, chief medical officer of the New York State Office of Mental Health (OMH), the nation's largest state mental health system, calls ACT teams "the most intensive and most expensive form of ambulatory care." They travel to wherever a person with SMI is, usually several times a week for a year or two, until their mental health is stabilized. Mobile teams can also provide an evaluation on the spot.

If you have to call the police because no mobile crisis team is available, explain to the dispatcher that your loved one has mental illness so that responding officers will be clear about the situation before they arrive. If possible, meet officers at the door, explaining where the person in crisis is, what behaviors they are exhibiting, and the cause for your concern. It's crucial to tell officers whether the person has access to anything that might be construed as a weapon. And here's another tip from Dr. Amador: "If your loved one has thrown or broken anything, don't try to clean up before the police come. Whatever damage your loved one has caused may be the only overt sign of illness the officers can see." Try to keep the interactions as cool and levelheaded as possible.

TIPS AND TRICKS TO HELP A LOVED ONE WITH CHRONIC, DEBILITATING SMI

From D. J. Jaffe, executive director of Mental
Illness Policy Org. and author of Insane Consequences:
How the Mental Health Industry Fails the Mentally Ill

- Pay someone, a friend, nurse, or responsible relative, to visit a loved one once a week to befriend them, take them shopping, out for a walk, or to the movies.

- Give your loved one gift certificates to local chain restaurants and stores in lieu of extra cash.

- Send care packages from your favorite online shops.

- Buy groceries online and have them delivered.

- Pay bills online to help ease their stress.

- Get a debit card that lets you control their expenses.

- Keep a single notebook with all of their medical paperwork, social security info, insurance numbers, medication list, and names and phone numbers of doctors so if they have to go to the ED or are admitted to the hospital, you can bring it along. Include a large, clear photo in case they ever go missing and you need one to give to police or show to neighbors and local establishments.

- Use your smartphone camera to photograph their ID, debit card, and Medicaid card (if applicable), and keep the photos on your phone for future reference.

- Get a HIPAA release to be able to talk to medical providers in language they'll respond to.

- Lay out medications in a weekly container.

- Try to get their inpatient doctor to take them on as an outpatient, too, to ensure continuity of care.

- Find a clubhouse program or start one in your community. One of the best examples of these is Fountain House in New York City, which offers day programs, vocational and educational training, supportive housing, and, most important, comradery and support without judgment.

- Move someplace with better services or where the person with SMI will feel more comfortable.

- Get your loved one out of the house and into their own space to reduce family tension. Or move to a home where they can have their own space with a separate entrance.

- If your loved one is homeless, leave clothing, toiletries, and snacks at their local hangouts.

- Get them a bright orange vest to protect them from getting hit by a car if they wander at night.

- Buy a companion dog, although you may have to watch over the pet's care.

- Provide love and understanding, find mutually agreeable goals, and reassure the person with SMI that they are good inside and out. And visit as much as possible.

For more tips, go to https://mentalillnesspolicy.org/coping.

FINDING A HEALTH CARE PROVIDER

As a clinical psychiatrist, I understand how hard it is to find a doctor, clinic, or hospital that you trust. Picking a provider is no easy task. Here are a few parameters to consider:

- **Treatment must be affordable:** Throwing money at the problems of SMI will not quickly resolve them. Mental illness is a war, not a battle. Although an expensive hospitalization may offer a diagnosis and be money well spent, it's important to conserve funds for long-term outpatient and inpatient care. Parity laws have enabled people with psychiatric conditions to receive benefits for outpatient and inpatient care comparable to folks with other medical issues. Even if you are dependent on state or federal health insurance plans, these are now legally required to offer psychiatric care in ways similar to medical care. We are far from realizing that goal of mental health parity for all Americans, but don't be deterred if your health care plan does not seem adequate. You can appeal any denials of care. For those who can afford it, policies that offer out-of-network coverage offer the most options. But whatever plan or coverage you have, think ahead to make sure that you can afford treatment for the long haul.

- **Find a provider with whom you have good chemistry:** Because of the lack of uniform treatment protocols, choosing the right psychiatrist, medical doctor, or nurse practitioner for medications and a psychiatrist, psychologist, social worker, or nurse for talk therapy may take some due diligence. Aside from making sure that your provider is affordable and convenient, you want someone who is well regarded by their peers and patients (as per word of mouth or in online reviews), is honest and ethical, and employs evidence-based best practices. You may want someone who works within a medical school or university setting and has colleagues looking over their shoulder. But most of all, as in any relationship, you want someone you can trust. You want *good chemistry*: an interpersonal fit, someone you can get along with, someone you can tell your truth to, to whom you can say nearly anything, and someone whose opinions you can respect.

- **Pick the treatment with the fewest side effects, but be open to all evidence-based options:** With all mental illnesses, from mild to the most severe, psychotherapy, or talk therapy, can change your brain for the better. Individual therapy, family therapy, group therapy, and self-help groups can make a world of difference. And unlike meds, no side effects!

- Medications are often required. Always seek the lowest dose and the least invasive treatment first as prescribed by a reputable, licensed clinician. Then, if lower medication doses are not sufficient or your talk therapy needs to be more intense and frequent, be ready to increase the level of care.

- Many of us make up our minds about what is acceptable and unacceptable without seeking out the latest scientific data. For instance, clozapine, an effective antipsychotic, is underused because of fears about its side effects. These concerns aren't unfounded, but such risks can be monitored and dosages moderated to find a balance for many patients who would otherwise suffer without the drug.

- Another maligned treatment is electroconvulsive therapy (ECT) because of its 1950s reputation. But, as used today, it's one of the safer and more effective treatments for entrenched depression that hasn't responded to other modalities. ECT helps up to 90 percent of patients with mood disorders.[6] Part of its bad reputation has to do with the nature of the treatment itself, and part with its sordid history. Until the 1960s, ECT was performed with electrodes placed on both sides of the head (making it more likely to cause memory problems) and without anesthesia (causing broken bones when patients flailed their bodies around during the therapeutic grand mal seizures that the treatment induced). Now, ECT is *always* done with anesthesia and is most often performed unilaterally, on one side of the head, on the nondominant hemisphere. No one would call the treatment pleasant, but it's nothing like the depiction in the 1975 film *One Flew over the Cuckoo's Nest*, which showed fictionalized versions of procedures conducted in the 1950s.

- **Self-care:** Too often we rely on the hour or so a week we may see a doctor or therapist, without thinking about what we can do in between appointments. Proper medical care is an essential piece of the puzzle, but it's no substitute for healthy living. Good nutrition, exercise, meditation, time with friends, proper sleep habits, laughter, cultivating a religious or spiritual life, and meaningful work and play can make a world of difference. Conversely, excessive alcohol use, taking recreational and unprescribed drugs, gambling, and other risky behaviors, as well as engaging in dysfunctional relationships—all of these may mess with your mind. Whether you are a patient or family member, self-care is crucial for your well-being.

USING THE LAW

We have discussed mental health courts (MHC), assisted outpatient treatment (AOT), and psychiatric advance directives (PAD)—all legal instruments to get the needed treatment. Each state and jurisdiction has its own forms, and these need to be filed through your local magistrate with the help of legal counsel.

Using the NAMI HelpLine and the listings on the Treatment Advocacy Center website (http://www.treatmentadvocacycenter .org), learn what legal resources are available in your state to pursue MHC, AOT, PAD, or health care powers of attorney. In many states, a PAD includes instructions about what a patient will consent to or refuse, while a power of attorney grants authority to a trusted loved one to make care decisions for someone who is incapable of doing so for themselves.

If you're the patient, a PAD specifies exactly what you want to have happen if you become psychotic or too impaired to make decisions. For family members, these directives can be particularly useful for fostering a sense of collaboration. Not only does one provide a crisis plan, it ensures the autonomy of the patient because they have put in writing how they want to be treated in the case of an emergency. This mitigates the alienation that many people with SMI experience both as a result of their own disordered thinking and by how they're treated by medical staff during a break with reality.

Although the experts I consulted confirmed the difficulty of enforcing such directives, they still recommended them as a valuable step in a constructive and collaborative conversation about care when one is in the throes of a psychotic episode. State-by-state guidelines and downloadable forms are available on the website of the National Resource Center on Psychiatric Advance Directives (https://www.nrc-pad.org).

SAMPLE ASSISTED OUTPATIENT TREATMENT (AOT) FORM

STATE OF NORTH CAROLINA Department of Health and Human Services
Division of Mental Health, Developmental Disabilities, and Substance Abuse Services

County _Durham_   File # _____

Client Record # _____

EXAMINATION AND RECOMMENDATION TO
DETERMINE
NECESSITY FOR INVOLUNTARY COMMITMENT

Film # _____

Name of Respondent: James Smith	Age 30	DOB 10-16-88	Sex M	Race C	M.S. single

Address (Street, Box Number, City, State, Zip (use facility address after 1 year in facility): 12 Mill St Durham NC 27710	County: Durham
	Phone: 919-555-1111

Legally Responsible Person ☐ Next of Kin (Name and Address) Eileen Smith	Relationship: wife
	Phone: 919-555-1111

Petitioner (Name and address)	Relationship:
	Phone

The above-named respondent was examined on _10-16_, 20_18_ at _2:30_ o'clock _P_.M. at _Durham Hospital_____, OR, I examined the respondent via telemedicine technology on _____, 20__ at _____ o'clock ___M. Included in the examination was an assessment of the respondent's: ☑ (1) current and previous mental illness or mental retardation including, if available, previous treatment history; (2) dangerousness to self or others as defined in G.S. 122C-3 (11*); (3) ability to survive safely without inpatient commitment, including the availability of supervision from family, friends, or others; and (4) capacity to make an informed decision concerning treatment. ☑ (1) current and previous substance abuse including, if available, previous treatment history; and (2) dangerousness to himself or others as defined in G.S. 122C-3 (11*). The following findings and recommendations are made based on this examination. For telemedicine evaluations only: ☐ I certify to a reasonable degree of medical certainty that the results of the examination via telemedicine were the same as if I had been personally present with the respondent OR ☐The respondent needs to be taken to a facility for a face to face evaluation. (*Statutory Definitions are on reverse side)

SECTION I – CRITERIA FOR COMMITMENT

Inpatient. It is my opinion that the respondent is:
(1st Exam – Physician or Psychologist)
(2nd Exam – Physician only)

☐ mentally ill; ☐ dangerous to self; ☐ dangerous to others
☐ in addition to being mentally ill is also mentally retarded
☐ none of the above

Outpatient. It is my opinion that:
(Physician or Psychologist)

☑ the respondent is mentally ill
☑ the respondent is capable of surviving safely in the community with available supervision
☑ based upon the respondent's treatment history, the respondent is in need of treatment in order to prevent further disability or deterioration which would predictably result in dangerousness as defined by G.S. 122C-3 (11*)
☑ the respondent's current mental status or the nature of his illness limits or negates his/her ability to make an informed decision to seek treatment voluntarily or comply with recommended treatment
☐ none of above

Substance Abuse. It is my opinion that the respondent is:
(1st Exam – Physician or Psychologist; 2nd Exam – If 1st exam done by Physician, 2nd exam may be done by Qual. Prof.)

☐ a substance abuser
☐ dangerous to himself or others
☐ none of the above

SECTION II – DESCRIPTION OF FINDINGS

Clear description of findings (findings for each criterion checked above in Section I must be described):

Mr. Smith has a long history of schizophrenia evidenced by delusions that he has super powers and can fly. In past he has jumped out of a building to fly when not on medication. He is currently not taking his medication and believes he can fly but wife says if he goes back on medication she can prevent (over) any harm.

Form No. DMH 5-72-01   EXAMINATION AND RECOMMENDATION FOR INVOLUNTARY COMMITMENT
Revised December 2009

Notable Physical Conditions:

None

Current Medications (medical and psychiatric)

Haloperidol D 50 mg
1 4 1x / month

Impression/Diagnosis:

Schizophrenia

SECTION III - RECOMMENDATION FOR DISPOSITION

☐ Inpatient Commitment for _____ days (respondent must be mentally ill **and** dangerous to self or others)

☑ Outpatient Commitment (respondent must meet **ALL** of the first four criteria outlined in Section I, **Outpatient**)
Proposed Outpatient Treatment Center or Physician: (Name) *Durham Mental Health Center*
(Address and Phone Number) *110 Main St*
Durham NC   919-555-1879

LME notified of appointment: (Name of LME and date) *Alliance Behavioral Health*

☐ Substance Abuse Commitment (respondent must meet both criteria outlined in Section I, **Substance Abuse**)
    ☐ Release respondent pending hearing - Referred to: _____
    ☐ Hold respondent at 24-hour facility pending hearing – Facility: _____

☐ Respondent does not meet the criteria for commitment but custody order states that the respondent was charged with a violent crime, including a crime involving assault with a deadly weapon, and that he was found not guilty by reason of insanity or incapable of proceeding: therefore, the respondent will not be released until so ordered following the court hearing.

☐ Respondent or Legally Responsible Person Consented to Voluntary Treatment

☐ Release Respondent and Terminate Proceedings (insufficient findings to indicate that respondent meets commitment criteria)

☐ Respondent was held 7 days from issuance of custody order but continues to meet commitment criteria. A new petition will be filed.

☐ Other (*Specify*) _____

Ronald Black M.D.	This is to certify that this is a true and exact copy of the Examination and Recommendation for Involuntary Commitment
Physician Signature	
Ronald Black MD	
Signature/Title – Eligible Psychologist/Qualified Professional	Original Signature – Record Custodian
Print Name of Examiner	
Durham Hospital	Title
Address or Facility	
Durham NC	Address or Facility
City and State	
919-555-1765	Date
Telephone Number	NOTE: Only copies to be introduced as evidence need to be certified

CC: Clerk of Superior Court where petition was initiated (initial hearing only)
Clerk of Superior Court where 24-hour facility is located or where outpatient treatment is supervised
Respondent or Respondent's Attorney and State's Attorneys, when applicable
Proposed Outpatient Treatment Center or Physician (Outpatient Commitment); Area Program / Physician (Substance Abuse Commitment)
NOTE: If it cannot be reasonably anticipated that the clerk will receive the copies within 48 hours of the time that it was signed, the physician or eligible psychologist/qualified professional shall communicate his findings to the clerk by telephone.

*STATUTORY DEFINITIONS
"Dangerous to self": Within the relevant past: (a) the individual has acted in such a way as to show: (1) that he would be unable without care, supervision, and the continued assistance of others not otherwise available, to exercise self-control, judgment, and discretion in the conduct of his daily responsibilities and social relations or to satisfy his need for nourishment, personal or medical care, shelter, or self-protection and safety; and (2) that there is a reasonable probability of his suffering serious physical debilitation within the near future unless adequate treatment is given. A showing of behavior that is grossly irrational, of actions that the individual is unable to control, of behavior that is grossly inappropriate to the situation, or of other evidence of severely impaired insight and judgment shall create a **prima facie** inference that the individual is unable to care for himself; or (b) the individual has attempted suicide or threatened suicide and that there is a reasonable probability of suicide unless adequate treatment is given; or (c) the individual has mutilated himself or attempted to mutilate himself and that there is a reasonable probability of serious self-mutilation unless adequate treatment is given. NOTE: Previous episodes of dangerousness to self, when applicable, may be considered when determining reasonable probability of physical debilitation, suicide, or self-mutilation.
"Dangerous to others": Within the relevant past, the individual has inflicted or attempted to inflict or threatened to inflict serious bodily harm on another, or has acted in such a way as to create a substantial risk of serious bodily harm to another, or has engaged in extreme destruction of property; and that there is a reasonable probability that this conduct will be repeated. Previous episodes of dangerousness to others, when applicable, may be considered when determining reasonable probability of future dangerous conduct.
"Mental illness": (a) when applied to an adult, an illness which so lessens the capacity of the individual to use self-control, judgment, and discretion in the conduct of his affairs and social relations as to make it necessary or advisable for him to be under treatment, care, supervision, guidance, or control; and (b) when applied to a minor, a mental condition, other than mental retardation alone, that so lessens or impairs the youth's capacity to exercise age adequate self-control and judgment in the conduct of his activities and social relationships so that he is in need of treatment.
"Substance abuser": An individual who engages in the pathological use or abuse of alcohol or other drugs in a way or to a degree that produces an impairment in personal, social, or occupational functioning. Substance abuse may include a pattern of tolerance and withdrawal.

SAMPLE PSYCHIATRIC ADVANCED DIRECTIVE (PAD) FORM

STATE OF NORTH CAROLINA

**ADVANCE INSTRUCTION FOR
MENTAL HEALTH TREATMENT**

COUNTY OF Durham

*(NOTICE TO PERSON MAKING AN INSTRUCTION FOR MENTAL HEALTH
TREATMENT)*

*This is an important legal document. It creates an instruction for mental health treatment. You
should consider filing it with the Advanced Health Care Directive Registry maintained by the
North Carolina Secretary of State: http://www.secretary.state.nc.us/ahcdr/thepage.aspx*

Before signing this document you should know these important facts:
*This document allows you to make decisions in advance about certain types of mental health
treatment. The instructions you include in this declaration will be followed if a physician or
eligible psychologist determines that you are incapable of making and communicating treatment
decisions. Otherwise, you will be considered capable to give or withhold consent for the
treatments. Your instructions may be overridden if you are being held in accordance with civil
commitment law. Under the Health Care Power of Attorney you may also appoint a person as
your health care agent to make treatment decisions for you if you become incapable. You have
the right to revoke this document at any time you have not been determined to be incapable.
YOU MAY NOT REVOKE THIS ADVANCE INSTRUCTION WHEN YOU ARE FOUND
INCAPABLE BY A PHYSICIAN OR OTHER AUTHORIZED MENTAL HEALTH TREATMENT
PROVIDER. A revocation is effective when it is communicated to your attending physician or
other provider. The physician or other provider shall note the revocation in your medical
record. To be valid, this advance instruction must be signed by two qualified witnesses,
personally known to you, who are present when you sign or acknowledge your signature. It must
also be acknowledged before a notary public.*

NOTICE TO PHYSICIAN OR OTHER MENTAL HEALTH TREATMENT PROVIDER
*Under North Carolina law, a person may use this advance instruction to provide consent for
future mental health treatment if the person later becomes incapable of making those decisions.
Under the Health Care Power of Attorney the person may also appoint a health care agent to
make mental health treatment decisions for the person when incapable. A person is "incapable"*

Page 1 of 8

when in the opinion of a physician or eligible psychologist the person currently lacks sufficient understanding or capacity to make and communicate mental health treatment decisions. This document becomes effective upon its proper execution and remains valid unless revoked. Upon being presented with this advance instruction, the physician or other provider must make it a part of the person's medical record. The attending physician or other mental health treatment provider must act in accordance with the statements expressed in the advance instruction when the person is determined to be incapable, unless compliance is not consistent with G.S. 122C-74(g). The physician or other mental health treatment provider shall promptly notify the principal and, if applicable, the health care agent, and document noncompliance with any part of an advance instruction in the principal's medical record. The physician or other mental health treatment provider may rely upon the authority of a signed, witnessed, dated and notarized advance instruction, as provided in G.S. 122C-75.

    I, <u>John Smith</u>, being an adult of sound mind, willfully and voluntarily make this advance instruction for mental health treatment to be followed if it is determined by a physician or eligible psychologist that my ability to receive and evaluate information effectively or communicate decisions is impaired to such an extent that I lack the capacity to refuse or consent to mental health treatment. "Mental health treatment" means the process of providing for the physical, emotional, psychological, and social needs of the principal. "Mental health treatment" includes electroconvulsive treatment (ECT), commonly referred to as "shock treatment," treatment of mental illness with psychotropic medication, and admission to and retention in a facility for care or treatment of mental illness.

    I understand that under G.S. 122C-57, other than for specific exceptions stated there, mental health treatment may not be administered without my express and informed written consent or, if I am incapable of giving my informed consent, the express and informed consent of my legally responsible person, my health care agent named pursuant to a valid health care power of attorney, or my consent expressed in this advance instruction for mental health treatment. I understand that I may become incapable of giving or withholding informed consent for mental treatment due to the symptoms of a diagnosed mental disorder. These symptoms may include: speaking very quickly, moving non-stop, not sleeping, not eating, expressing grandiose thoughts, believing I have special powers, irritability, irrational beliefs—such as that I am a powerful politician.

PSYCHOACTIVE MEDICATIONS

If I become incapable of giving or withholding informed consent for mental health treatment, my instructions regarding psychoactive medications are as follows: *(Place initials beside choice.)*

__JS____   I consent to the administration of the following medications: <u>lithium, Depakote, aripiprazole,</u>

__JS_   I do not consent to the administration of the following medications: <u>haloperidol</u>

Conditions or limitations: <u>haloperidol makes me restless and stiff</u>

ADMISSION TO AND RETENTION IN FACILITY

If I become incapable of giving or withholding informed consent for mental health treatment, my instructions regarding admission to and retention in a health care facility for mental health treatment are as follows: *(Place initials beside choice.)*

__JS____   I consent to being admitted to a health care facility for mental health treatment. My facility preference is <u>Durham Hospital</u>. Sandford Hospital

_____   I do not consent to being admitted to a health care facility for mental health treatment.

This advance instruction cannot, by law, provide consent to retain me in a facility for more than ten (10) days.

Conditions or limitations: I do not want to go to a hospital more than an hour from my home.

ADDITIONAL INSTRUCTIONS

These instructions shall apply during the entire length of my incapacity. In case of mental health crisis, please contact:

1.   Name: <u>Jill Smith</u>

     Home Address: <u>11 Smith Guest Road, Durham, NC</u>

     Home Telephone Number: <u>919-555-0303</u>

     Work Telephone Number: <u>919-555-0303</u>

     Relationship to Me: <u>wife</u>

2.   Name: <u>Bob Smith</u>

     Home Address: <u>11 Smith Guest Road, Durham NC</u>

     Home Telephone Number: <u>919-555-0303</u>

Work Telephone Number: <u>919-555-0303</u>

Relationship to Me: son

3.! My Physician:

Name: <u>Ralph Brown, MD</u>

Telephone Number: <u>919-555-6767</u>

4.! My Therapist:

Name: <u>same</u>

Telephone Number: same

The following may cause me to experience a mental health crisis: <u>Losing my job, not sleeping,</u> <u>fighting with my family, not taking my medications.</u>

The following help me avoid a hospitalization: <u>Taking my medications, scheduling extra</u> <u>sessions with my doctor with my wife. Getting exercise when stressed out.</u>

I generally react to being hospitalized as follows: I can be very cooperative and calm as long as my wife accompanies me and the nurses and doctors treat me respectfully.

Staff of the hospital or crisis unit can help me by doing the following: Give me my medications as needed. Find a quiet place for me. Keep me away from agitated patients. Speak quietly and respectfully to me.

I give permission for the following person or people to visit me: Any member of my family or others that my wife suggests.

Instructions concerning any other medical interventions, such as electroconvulsive (ECT) treatment (commonly referred to as "shock treatment": <u>If my outpatient doctor and wife</u> <u>recommend ECT I give my permission to administer it. ECT team must be well experienced.</u>

Other instructions:

<u>Please make sure my wife gives consent to any medications, tests, or procedures and that she has</u> <u>consulted with my outpatient doctor.</u>

_____ *(Initial if applicable)* I have attached an additional sheet of instructions to be followed and considered part of this advance instruction.

SHARING OF INFORMATION BY PROVIDERS

I understand that the information in this document may be shared by my mental health treatment provider with any other mental health treatment provider who may serve me when necessary to provide treatment in accordance with this advance instruction.

Other instructions about sharing of information: <u>Please share this information with my primary care physician.</u>

SIGNATURE OF PRINCIPAL

By signing here, I indicate that I am mentally alert and competent, fully informed as to the contents of this document, and understand the full impact of having made this advance instruction for mental health treatment.

_____10-16-18_____	_____XXX_____
Date	Signature of Principal

NATURE OF WITNESSES

I hereby state that the principal is personally known to me, that the principal signed or acknowledged the principal's signature on this advance instruction for mental health treatment in my presence, that the principal appears to be of sound mind and not under duress, fraud, or undue influence, and that I am not:

a.! The attending physician or mental health service provider or an employee of the physician or mental health treatment provider;

b.! An owner, operator, or employee of an owner or operator of a health care facility in which the principal is a patient or resident; or

c.! Related within the third degree to the principal or to the principal's spouse.

Page 6 of 8

AFFIRMATION OF WITNESS

We affirm that the principal is personally known to us, that the principal signed or acknowledged the principal's signature on this advance instruction for mental health treatment in our presence, that the principal appears to be of sound mind and not under duress, fraud, or undue influence, and that neither of us is:

a.! A person appointed as an attorney-in-fact by this document;

b.! The principal's attending physician or mental health service provider or a relative of the physician or provider;

c.! The owner, operator, or relative of an owner or operator of a facility in which the principal is a patient or resident; or

d.! A person related to the principal by blood, marriage, or adoption.

Witnessed by:

Liz Apple _____   Steve Moon _____

Witness   Witness
10-16-18 _____   10-16-18 _____
Date   Date

STATE OF NORTH CAROLINA

COUNTY OF <u>Durham</u>

CERTIFICATION OF NOTARY PUBLIC

I, <u>Ron Brown</u>, a Notary Public for the County cited above in the State of North Carolina, hereby certify that <u>John Smith</u> appeared before me and swore or affirmed to me and to the witnesses in my presence that this instrument is an advance instruction for mental health treatment, and that he/she willingly and voluntarily made and executed it as his/her free act and deed for the purposes expressed in it.

I further certify that <u>Liz Apple</u> and <u>Steve Moon</u>, witnesses, appeared before me and swore or affirmed that they witnessed <u>John Smith</u> sign the attached advance instruction for mental health treatment, believing him/her to be of sound mind; and also swore that at the time they witnessed the signing they were not (i) the attending physician or mental health treatment provider or an employee of the physician or mental health treatment provider and (ii) they were not an owner, operator, or employee of an owner or operator of a health care facility in which the principal is a patient or resident, and (iii) they were not related within the third degree to the principal or to the principal's spouse. I further certify that I am satisfied as to the genuineness and due execution of the instrument.

This the <u>16</u> day of <u>10</u>, 20<u>18</u>.

<u>Ron Brown</u>
Notary Public
My Commission Expires:10-16-2020

These sample documents were supplied by one of the nation's leading experts on PAD and AOT, Dr. Marvin Swartz. They should not be construed as legal or medical advice, which you should seek before embarking on any patient plan, particularly one that involves directives for medical care. Dr. Swartz also filled out sample forms on a hypothetical patient for assisted outpatient treatment (AOT).

....

WHAT TO FIGHT FOR

Any concerned citizen needs to be aware of the societal changes that must take place before we can call this an equal society for all. Here is a quick summary of the policy changes that I urge you to support:

- Improve access to care: Create a health care delivery system that favors evidence-based scientific treatments being delivered in the community or outpatient care while dramatically increasing the current number of inpatient treatment beds for mental illness care.

- Improve aftercare: Embrace comprehensive wraparound approaches that include housing, support, health and wellness, and access to decent housing, vocational opportunities, and opportunities for socialization and growth.

- Support increased training of first responders: Increase crisis intervention training for police and other first responders to foster compassionate treatment instead of imprisonment or punishment.

- Decriminalize mental illness: Promote decarceration (decriminalization) of people with mental illness with judicial reforms such as mental health courts to divert people from jail, and address institutionalized prejudice and racism, which foster incarceration versus treatment.

- Fair and equitable care: Prioritize services based on who is sickest, not who can pay, and support legislation that creates parity of mental health services on par with medical and surgical care.

- Models of care endorsed by people with SMI: Include people with mental illness in our dialogue about treatment and social reform rather than shutting them out with an attitude of *they don't know what's good for them.*

- Address substance abuse: Focus on the role of substance abuse— itself a life-threatening disorder—which is preventable and treatable and complicates and contributes to serious mental disorders such as depression, bipolar disorder, and schizophrenia.

- It's all about finding good treatments: Expand and improve scientific research because the best solutions are prevention and cure.

If you're interested in reading publications about social policy issues, please see: https://www.scattergoodfoundation.org/think/publications/policy-paper-series/.

ACKNOWLEDGMENTS

I stand on the shoulders of giants. Aside from those listed in the Author's Note and those I mentioned in the book, I am indebted to Michael Donaldson, Dr. Jeff Geller, Dr. Christina Ghaly, Julio Lagos, Drew Patrick, Dr. Mitchell Katz, Thomas Bena, Dr. Marcia Goin, Diana Barrett, Sheila Leddy, Mark Anthony Johnson, Geanne Belton, Kristina Bicher, Linda Rosenberg, George Crawford, Dr. Chris Barley, Cynthia and Rob Doyle, Dr. Charles Silberstein, Laura Roosevelt, Dr. Peter Kramer, Barbara Ricci, Shirley Perlman, Don Santel, Kelly McGinnis, Dr. Matt Biel, Dr. Peter Finklestein, Issac Hager, Noah Ward, John Cheng, Fred Wong, Lisa Tawil, Lindsay Gordon, Casey Maloney, Lauren Pabst, Megan Ryan, Christine Machese, Annie Roney, Mimi McKay, Peter Reineker, Sara Bernstein, Ed Morrissey, Matt O'Neil, Jon Alpert, Sheila Nevins, Geof Bartz, Nancy Abraham, Chuck Harman, Dr. Ken Duckworth, Keith Arnold, Gabe Grimalt, William Morrison, Jason Campbell, Valerie Marcus, Dr. Phillip Wilner, Dr. Eslee Samberg, Celia Maria Freitas, Martin Sherry, Joe Pyle, Rick Kellar, Patty Quillin, Mark and Stephanie Robinson, Francis Greenburger, Sam Decker, Jeff Berzon, Paul Finegan, Peter Kenney. I am immeasurably grateful for guidance and support from Alexander and Claire Rosenberg; Lynn Novick; Todd and Bette Sacktor; Robert, Andrew, Todd, and David Zitin; Bruce and Ellen Roseman; Hedy, Ivan, Robert, and Eddy Taub; Neil Schwartz; Dr. Roy Goldberg; Dr. David W. Preven; Judith Sarafini-Sauli; Florence and Maya van Putten; and Nate, Norman, Bill, Sam, and Ruthie Rosenberg.

This work has been made possible through sponsorship from the Independent Television Service, Public Broadcasting Service, Corporation for Public

Broadcasting, John D. and Catherine T. MacArthur Foundation Journalism and Media Program, International Documentary Association, Fiduciary Fund, Fledgling Fund, PEGS, Scattergood Foundation, Meadow Fund, Towers Family Fund, the Sundance Institute and Film Festival, and through the support of Avery Publishing (an imprint or Penguin Random House) and their team under the direction of Megan Newman.

The people to whom I am most grateful are the patients, their families, and their health care providers. They shared their stories for no purpose other than to prevent the suffering of others. They inspire me every day.

NOTES

INTRODUCTION

1. National Institute of Mental Health. *Mental Illness.* Washington, DC: U.S. Department of Health and Human Services, February 2019. Retrieved from www.nimh.nih.gov/health/statistics/mental-illness.shtml

2. *Ibid.*

3. Merikangas, K. R., and V. L. McClair. "Epidemiology of Substance Use Disorders." *Human Genetics* 131, no. 5 (2012): 779–89. Retrieved from https:// www.ncbi.nlm.nih.gov/pmc/articles/PMC4408274/

4. Interdepartmental Serious Mental Illness Coordinating Committee. *The Way Forward: Federal Action for a System That Works for All People Living with SMI and SED and Their Families and Caregivers.* Report to Congress. December 13, 2017. Retrieved from https://www.samhsa.gov/sites/default /files/programs_campaigns/ismicc_2017_report_to_congress.pdf

5. *Ibid.*

6. 1993 *Federal Register.* Notice 58 FR 29425, May 20, 1993. Cited in Committee on National Statistics. *Measuring Serious Emotional Disturbance in Children: Workshop Summary.* Washington, DC: National Academies Press, January 28, 2016. Available from www.ncbi.nlm.nih.gov/books /NBK368053/

7. In 2016, Emma McGinty and colleagues compared news media stories concerning mental illness for 1995–2004 and 2005–2014. The number of stories in which stigma or discrimination was mentioned as a problem increased from 23 percent in 1995–2004 to 28 percent in 2005–2014. McGinty, E. E., A. Kennedy-Hendricks, S. Choksy, and C. L. Barry. "Trends in News Media Coverage of Mental Illness in the United States: 1995–2014." *Health Affairs* 35, no. 6 (2016): 1121–29.

8. Baker, P., and M. Haberman. "Anthony Scaramucci's Uncensored Rant: Foul Words and Threats to Have Priebus Fired." *New York Times.* July 27, 2017. Retrieved from www.nytimes.com/2017/07/27/us/politics /scaramucci-priebus-leaks.html

CHAPTER I: HOW IT ALL BEGAN

1. Department of Housing and Urban Development. *The 2018 Annual Homeless Assessment Report to Congress.* Washington, DC. 2018. Retrieved

from https://www.hudexchange.info/resources/documents/2018-AHAR
-Part-1.pdf

2. Porter, R. *Mind-Forg' d Manacles: A History of Madness in England from
the Restoration to the Regency*. Cambridge: Harvard University Press, 1987,
p. 122.

3. César de Saussure. *A Foreign View of England in the Reigns of George
I and George II: The Letters of Monsieur César de Saussure to His Family*.
Translated and edited by Madame Van Muyden. Cited in Porter, *Mind-
Forg'd Manacles*, p. 126.

4. Andrews, J., A. Briggs, R. Porter, P. Tucker, and K. Waddington. *The
History of Bethlem*. London: Routledge, 1997, p. 36.

5. Porter, *Mind-Forg'd Manacles*, p. 123.

6. *Ibid.*, p. 128.

7. Andrews et al., *The History of Bethlem*, p. 114.

8. U.S. National Library of Medicine. *Diseases of the Mind: Highlights of
American Psychiatry Through 1900—Early Psychiatric Hospitals and Asylums*.
Washington, DC: National Institutes of Health, January 18, 2017. Retrieved
from www.nlm.nih.gov/hmd/diseases/early.html

9. Grob, G. N., and H. H. Goldman. *The Dilemma of Federal Mental Health
Policy: Radical Reform or Incremental Change?* New Brunswick, NJ: Rutgers
University Press, 2006, p. 3.

10. Dix, D. L. *Memorial to the Legislature of Massachusetts, 1843*. Boston:
Munroe & Francis, 1843, p. 4. Quoted in Grob and Goldman, *The Dilemma
of Federal Mental Health Policy*, p. 3.

11. *Ibid.*

12. *Ibid.*, p. 4.

13. Gamwell, L., and N. Tomes. *Madness in America: Cultural and Medical
Perceptions of Mental Illness Before 1914*. Binghamton, NY: Cornell
University Press, 1995, p. 42.

14. *Ibid.*, p. 41.

15. *Ibid.*, pp. 38–39.

16. Rocos, B., and T. J. Chesser. "Injuries in Jumpers: Are There Any
Patterns?" *World Journal of Orthopedics* 7, no. 3 (March 18, 2016): 182–87.
Retrieved from doi: 10.5312/wjo.v7.i3.182.

17. *Ibid.*

18. Treatment Advocacy Center. Dr. E. Fuller Torrey Talks About His
Loved One. YouTube video, June 14, 2012. Retrieved from www.youtube
.com/watch?v=bWX13jlVL0k

19. *Ibid.*

20. *Ibid.*

21. Johnston, J. "The Ghost of the Schizophrenogenic Mother." *Virtual Mentor* 15, no. 9 (2013): 801–5. Retrieved from https://journalofethics .ama-assn.org/article/ghost-schizophrenogenic-mother/2013-09

22. Mencimer, Stephanie. "Dr. E. Fuller Torrey: Washington City Paper Profile," Mental Illness Policy Org., January 16, 1998, http://mentalillness policy.org/media/eft/torrey-bio-dc-paper.html

23. Treatment Advocacy Center. *Who We Are and What We Do* (n.d.). Retrieved from https://www.treatmentadvocacycenter.org/about-us

24. Valenstein, E. S. *Great and Desperate Cures: The Rise and Decline of Psychosurgery and Other Radical Treatments for Mental Illness.* New York: Basic Books, 2015.

25. E. Fuller Torrey (2014). *American Psychosis.* (p. 4). New York, NY: Oxford University Press.

26. Goodwin, Doris Kearns. *The Fitzgeralds and the Kennedys: An American Saga.* New York: St. Martin's Press, 1987, p. 741. Quoted in E. Fuller Torrey, *American Psychosis: How the Federal Government Destroyed the Mental Illness Treatment System.* Oxford: Oxford University Press, p. 8.

27. *Ibid.*

28. Kessler, Ronald. *The Sins of the Father: Joseph P. Kennedy and the Dynasty He Founded.* New York: Warner Books, 1996, pp. 242–46. Quoted in Torrey, *American Psychosis*, p. 12.

29. *Ibid.*, p. 255.

30. Torrey, *American Psychosis*, p. 19.

31. Felix, R. H. (1948). "Mental Hygiene and Public Health." *American Journal of Orthopsychiatry* 18, no. 4 (1948): 679–84. Quoted in Torrey, American Psychosis, p. 25.

32. Foley H. A., and S. S. Sharfstein. *Madness and Government: Who Cares for the Mentally Ill?* Washington, DC: American Psychiatric Press, 1983, p. 29; Beer, S. H. "Foreword." In H. A. Foley, *Community Mental Health Legislation: The Formative Process.* Lexington, MA: Lexington Books, 1975, p. xi. Quoted in Torrey, *American Psychosis*, p. 26.

33. Ban, T. A. (2007). "Fifty Years Chlorpromazine: An Historical Perspective." *Neuropsychiatric Disease and Treatment* 3, no. 4 (2007): 495–500.

34. Grob and Goldman, *Dilemma of Federal Mental Health Policy*, viii.

35. Kennedy, J. F. (1963, February 5). "Special Message to the Congress on

Mental Illness and Mental Retardation." February 5, 1963. In G. Peters and J. T. Woolley, *The American Presidency Project*. Retrieved from http://www .presidency.ucsb.edu/ws/?pid=9546

36. *Ibid.*

37. *Ibid.*

38. Grob and Goldman, *Dilemma of Federal Mental Health Policy*, p. vii.

39. Grob, G. N. *The Mad Among Us: A History of the Care of America's Mentally Ill*. New York: Free Press, 1994, pp. 234–35 and 261. Quoted in E. E. McGinty et al. (2018). "Communicating About Mental Illness and Violence: Balancing Stigma and Increased Support for Services." *Journal of Health Politics, Policy and Law* 43, no. 2 (2018): 185–28. Retrieved from, https://doi.org/10.1215/03616878-4303507

40. Frank, Richard G., and Sherry A. Glied. *Better But Not Well: Mental Health Policy in the United States Since 1950*. Baltimore: Johns Hopkins University Press, 2006, p. 54.

41. Torrey, *American Psychosis*, p. 33.

42. Gronfein, W. (1985). "Psychotropic Drugs and the Origins of Deinstitu-tionalization." *Social Problems* 32, no. 5 (1985): 437–54. Quoted in Torrey, *American Psychosis*, p. 33.

43. Holland, G. "LA's Homelessness Surged 75% in Six Years. Here's Why the Crisis Has Been Decades in the Making." *Los Angeles Times*, February 1, 2018. Retrieved from https://www.latimes.com/local/lanow/la-me-homeless -how-we-got-here-20180201-story.html

44. Los Angeles Homeless Services Authority. *Homelessness in LA County*. 2018. Retrieved from https://lafh.org/2018-homeless-count

CHAPTER 2: ME-TOO MEDICINES

1. HOK. Los Angeles County and University of Southern California Medical Center. *HOK*. No date. Retrieved from www.hok.com/design/type /healthcare/los-angeles-county-university-of-southern-california-medical -center/; (n.d.). Los Angeles County and University of Southern California Medical Center. *Architizer*. No date. Retrieved from architizer.com/projects /lac-usc-medical-center

2. Daumit, G. L., F. B. Dickerson, N.-Y. Wang, A. Dalcin, G. J. Jerome, C. A. M. Anderson, et al. "A Behavioral Weight-Loss Intervention in Persons with Serious Mental Illness." *New England Journal of Medicine* 368, no. 17 (2013): 1594–602. Retrieved from https://www.ncbi.nlm.nih.gov /pubmed/23517118

3. Olfson, M., T. Gerhard, C. Huang, S. Crystal, and T. S. Stroup. "Premature Mortality Among Adults with Schizophrenia in the United States." *JAMA Psychiatry* 72, no. 12 (2015): 1172–81. Retrieved from https://www.ncbi.nlm.nih.gov/pubmed/26509694; Hayes, J. F., L. Marston, K. Walters, M. B. King, and D. P. J. Osborn. "Mortality Gap for People with Bipolar Disorder and Schizophrenia: UK-Based Cohort Study 2000–2014." *British Journal of Psychiatry* 211, no. 3 (2017): 175–81. Retrieved from https://www.ncbi.nlm.nih.gov/pubmed/28684403

4. Crilly, J. "The History of Clozapine and Its Emergence in the US Market: A Review and Analysis." *History of Psychiatry* 18, no. 1 (2007): 57. Retrieved from https://www.ncbi.nlm.nih.gov/pubmed/17580753

5. Glied and Frank, *Better But Not Well*, p. 29.

6. *Ibid.*

7. Geddes, J. R. "Atypical Antipsychotics in the Treatment of Schizophrenia: Systematic Review, Metaregression and Evidence-Based Treatment Recommendations." *Schizophrenia Research* 41, no. 1 (2000): 1371–76. Retrieved from doi:10.1016/s0920-9964(00)90384-0; Lieberman, J. A. "Comparative Efficacy and Safety of Atypical and Conventional Antipsychotic Drugs in First-Episode Psychosis: A Randomized, Double-Blind Trial of Olanzapine Versus Haloperidol." *American Journal of Psychiatry* 160, no. 8 (2003): 1396–1404. Retrieved from doi:10.1176/appi.ajp.160.8.1396. Quoted in Glied and Frank, *Better But Not Well*, pp. 30–31.

8. Scherk, H., F. G. Pajonk, and S. Leucht. "Second-Generation Antipsychotic Agents in the Treatment of Acute Mania: A Systematic Review and Metaanalysis of Randomized Control Trials." *JAMA Psychiatry* 64, no. 4 (2007): 442–55. Retrieved from https://jamanetwork.com/journals/jamapsychiatry/fullarticle/209997

9. Sussman, N. "Review of Atypical Antipsychotics and Weight Gain." *Journal of Clinical Psychiatry* 62 (2001): 5–12. Retrieved from www.ncbi.nlm.nih.gov/pubmed/11603886

10. Higgins, E. S. "Is Mental Health Declining in the U.S.?" *Scientific American*, January 1, 2017. Retrieved from https://www.scientificamerican.com/article/is-mental-health-declining-in-the-u-s/

11. Meltzer, H. Y. "Treatment-Resistant Schizophrenia—the Role of Clozapine." *Current Medical Research and Opinion* 14, no. 1 (1997): 1–20.

12, Crilly, J. "The History of Clozapine and Its Emergence in the US Market." *History of Psychiatry* 18, no.1 (2007): 57. Retrieved from doi:10.1177/0957154x07070335

13. Alvir, J. M., J. A. Lieberman, A. Z. Safferman, J. L. Schwimmer, and J. A. Schaaf. "Clozapine-Induced Agranulocytosis. Incidence and Risk Factors in the United States." *New England Journal of Medicine* 329, no. 3 (1993): 162–67. Retrieved from https://www.ncbi.nlm.nih.gov/pubmed/8515788

CHAPTER 3: DUNGEONS AND DRAGONS: CRIMINALIZING MENTAL ILLNESS

1. Khan-Cullors, P., and A. Bandele. *When They Call You A Terrorist: A Black Lives Matter Memoir.* New York: St. Martin's Press, 2017, p. 50.

2. *Ibid.*, p. 50.

3. Roth, A. *Insane: America's Criminal Treatment of Mental Illness.* New York: Basic Books, 2018, pp. 52–53.

4. Chapter 3: "Mental Health Care for African Americans. In Office of the Surgeon General, *Mental Health: Culture, Race, and Ethnicity: A Supplement to Mental Health. A Report to the Surgeon General.* Rockville, MD: Substance Abuse and Mental Health Services Administration, 2001. Retrieved from https:// www.ncbi.nlm.nih.gov/books/NBK44251/

5. Strakowski, S. M., S. L. McElroy, P. E. Keck, and S. A. West. "Racial Influence on Diagnosis in Psychotic Mania." *Journal of Affective Disorders* 39, no. 2 (1996): 157–62. Retrieved from https://www.sciencedirect.com /science/article/pii/0165032796000286

6. Levin, A. "Racism Lingers in Mental Health System." *Psychiatric News,* November 8, 2013. Retrieved from https://doi.org/10.1176/appi.pn.2013 .11b16

7. *Ibid.*

8. Saleh, A. Z., P. S. Appelbaum, X. Liu, T. S. Stroup, and M. Wall. (2018). "Deaths of People with Mental Illness During Interactions with Law Enforce ment." *International Journal of Law and Psychiatry* 58 (2018): 110–16. Retrieved from https://www.sciencedirect.com/science/article/abs /pii/S0160252717301954

9. *Ibid.*

10. Treatment Advocacy Center. *Road Runners: The Role and Impact of Law Enforcement in Transporting Individuals with Severe Mental Illness.* Arlington, VA, 2019.

11. *Ibid.*

12. "Fatal Force." *Washington Post,* March 31, 2019. Retrieved from https:// www.washingtonpost.com/graphics/2018/national/police-shootings-2018 /?utm_term=.feaf86fb5426

13. Harki, G. A. (2018, August 23). "Horrific Deaths, Brutal Treatment: Mental Illness in America's Jails." *Virginian-Pilot*, August 23, 2018. Retrieved from https://pilotonline.com/news/local/projects/jail-crisis /article_5ba8a112-974e-11e8-ba17-b734814f14db.html

14. Roth, *Insane*, p. 44.

15. Torrey, E. F., M. T. Zdanowicz, A. D. Kennard, H. R. Lamb, D. F. Eslinger, M. C. Biasotti, et al. *The Treatment of Persons with Mental Illness in Prisons and Jails: A State Survey*. Arlington, VA: Treatment Advocacy Center, 2014. Retrieved from https://www.treatmentadvocacycenter.org/storage /documents/treatment-behind-bars/treatment-behind-bars.pdf

16. *Serious Mental Illness Prevalence in Jails and Prisons*. Arlington, VA: Treatment Advocacy Center, n.d. Retrieved from www.treatment advocacycenter.org/evidence-and-research/learn-more-about/3695

17. Roth, *Insane*, pp. 40–41.

18. Winerip, M., and M. Schirtz. "Rikers: Where Mental Illness Meets Brutality in Jail. *New York Times*, July 14, 2014. Retrieved from https:// www.nytimes.com/2014/07/14/nyregion/rikers-study-finds-prisoners -injured-by-employees.html?module=inline

19. Torrey et al., *The Treatment of Persons with Mental Illness in Prisons and Jails*, p. 118.

20. *Ibid.*, p. 119.

21. *CIT Map*. Memphis, TN: University of Memphis CIT Center, n.d. Retrieved from http://cit.memphis.edu/citmap/

22. Goldman, S. "In New York, an Influential First Lady Redefines the Position." *New York Times*, October 20, 2017. Retrieved from https://www.nytimes .com/2017/10/20/nyregion/chirlane-mccray-first-lady-de-blasio.html

23. For more information about mental health first aid, see https://www.nydaily news.com/opinion/ny-oped-the-sane-way-to-attack-mental-illness-20190307 -story.html and thenationalcouncil.org/about/mental-health -first-aid/

24. Torrey et al., *The Treatment of Persons with Mental Illness in Prisons and Jails*. Retrieved from https://www.treatmentadvocacycenter.org/storage /documents/treatment-behind-bars/treatment-behind-bars.pdf

CHAPTER 4: THROWAWAY PEOPLE

1. *ACEP Emergency Department Violence Poll Research Results*. Washington, DC: American College of Emergency Physicians, September 2018. Retrieved from newsroom.acep.org/download/2018ACEP+Emergency+ Department+ Violence+PollResults.pdfcite

2. Leo, J. (2006). "Schizophrenia Adoption Studies." *PLoS Medicine* 3, no. 8 (2006).

3. Fischer, M. "Psychoses in the Offspring of Schizophrenic Monozygotic Twins and Their Normal Co-twins." *British Journal of Psychiatry* 118, no. 542 (1971): 43–52; Cardno, A. G., E. J. Marshall, B. Coid, A. M. Macdonald, T. R. Ribchester, N. J. Davies, et al. "Heritability Estimates for Psychotic Disorders: The Maudsley Twin Psychosis Series." *Archives of General Psychiatry* 56, no. 2 (1999): 162–68.

4. Kendler, K. S., and A. M. Gruenberg, A. M. "An Independent Analysis of the Danish Adoption Study of Schizophrenia. VI: The Relationship Between Psychiatric Disorders as Defined by DSM-III in the Relatives and Adoptees." *Archives of General Psychiatry* 41, no. 6 (June 1984): 555–64. Retrieved from https://jamanetwork.com/journals/jamapsychiatry/article-abstract/493347; Hilker, Rikke, et al. "Heritability of Schizophrenia and Schizophrenia Spectrum Based on the Nationwide Danish Twin Register." *Biological Psychiatry* 83, no. 6: 492–498.

5. The Brainstorm Consortium. "Analysis of Shared Heritability in Common Disorders of the Brain." *Science* 360, no. 6395 (June 22, 2018). Retrieved from doi:10.1126/science.aap8757

6. Clark, E. G., and N. Danbolt. "The Oslo Study of the Natural Course of Untreated Syphilis." *Medical Clinics of North America* 48 (1964): 613–21.

7. Torrey E. F., R. Rawlings, and R. H. Yolken. (2000). "The Antecedents of Psychoses: A Case-Control Study of Selected Risk Factors." *Schizophrenia Research* 46, no. 1 (2000): 17–23.

8. Dickerson, F. B., C. Stallings, A. Origoni, E. Katsafanas, C. L. G. Savage, A. B. Schweinfurth, et al. "Effect of Probiotic Supplementation on Schizophrenia Symptoms and Association with Gastrointestinal Functioning: A Randomized, Placebo-Controlled Trial." *Primary Care Companion for CNS Disorders* 16, no. 1 (2014). Retrieved from https://www.ncbi.nlm.nih.gov/pmc/articles/PMC4048142/

9. Sekar, A., A. R. Bialas, H. de Rivera, A. Davis, T. R. Hammond, N. Kamitaki, et al. (2016). "Schizophrenia Risk from Complex Variation of Complement Component 4." *Nature* 530, no. 7589 (2016): 177–83. Retrieved from https://www.ncbi.nlm.nih.gov/pmc/articles/PMC4752392/

10. Tamminga, C. A., and D. R. Medoff. (2000). "The Biology of Schizophrenia." *Dialogues Clinical Neuroscience* 2, no. 4 (2000): 339–48; Kim, Y., R. Santos, F. H. Gage, and M. C. Marchetto. "Molecular Mechanisms of Bipolar Disorder: Progress Made and Future Challenges."

Frontiers in Cellular Neuroscience 11, no. 30 (2017). Retrieved from doi:10.3389/fncel.2017.00030

11. Bremmer, J. D. (1999). "Does Stress Damage the Brain?" *Biological Psychiatry* 45, no. 7 (1999): 797–805. Retrieved from https://www.ncbi .nlm.nih.gov/pubmed/10202566

12. Draine, J., M. S. Salzer, D. P. Culhane, and T. R. Hadley. "Role of Social Disadvantage in Crime, Joblessness, and Homelessness Among Persons with Serious Mental Illness." *Psychiatric Services* 53, no. 5 (2002): 565–73. Retrieved from https://doi.org/10.1176/appi.ps.53.5.565

13. Dixon, L., G. Haas, R. Duilt, P. Weiden, J. Sweeney, and D. Hien. (1989). "Schizophrenia and Substance Abuse: Preferences, Predictors and Psychopathology." *Schizophrenia Research* 2, nos. 1–2 (1989): 6. Retrieved from https:// doi.org/10.1016/0920-9964(89)90042-X

14. *Serious Mental Illness and Homelessness*. Arlington, VA: Treatment Advocacy Center, 2016. Retrieved from https://www.treatmentadvoca cycenter.org/storage/documents/backgrounders/smi-and-homelessness.pdf

15. *Common Comorbidities with Substance Use Disorders*. National Institute on Drug Abuse, n.d. Retrieved from https://www.drugabuse.gov/publications /research-reports/common-comorbidities-substance-use-disorders/part-1 -connection-between-substance-use-disorders-mental-illness

16. *Homelessness in LA County*. Los Angeles Homeless Services Authority, 2018. Retrieved from https://lafh.org/2018-homeless-count

CHAPTER 5: "MY SON DIED WITH HIS CIVIL LIBERTIES INTACT"

1. *Promoting Assisted Outpatient Treatment*. Arlington, VA: Treatment Advocacy Center, n.d. Retrieved from https://www.treatmentadvocacy center.org/fixing-the-system/promoting-assisted-outpatient-treatment

2. *Program Statistics: Petitions Filed*. Database. Albany, NY: New York State Office of Mental Health, 2019. Retrieved from https://my.omh.ny.gov /analytics/saw.dll?dashboard#reports

3. Gorman, C. "The System Is Failing the Mentally Ill—Not the Cops." *New York Post*, August 14, 2018. Retrieved from nypost.com/2018/08/14 /the-system-is-failing-the-mentally-ill-not-the-cops/

4. *Grading the States: An Analysis of Involuntary Psychiatric Treatment Laws*. Arlington, VA: Treatment Advocacy Center, 2018. Retrieved from https:// www.treatmentadvocacycenter.org/grading-the-states

5. *Kendra's Law: Final Report on the Status of Assisted Outpatient Treatment*.

Albany, NY: New York State Office of Mental Health, 2005; Hauert, A., E. Johnson, N. Kirpalani, J. Martin, and D. Miller. (2012). "The Cost of Healthcare: Does More Care = Better Care?" *Perspectives* 8.

6. Health Management Associates. *State and Community Considerations for Demonstrating the Cost-Effectiveness of AOT Services.* Arlington, VA: Treatment Advocacy Center, 2015.

7. Swanson, J., E. E. McGinty, S. Fazel, and V. Mays. "Mental Illness and Reduction of Gun Violence and Suicide: Bringing Epidemiological Research to Policy." *Annals of Epidemiology* 25, no. 5 (2014): 366–76.

8. Swartz, M. S., J. W. Swanson, H. R. Wagner, B. J. Burns, V. A. Hiday, and R. Borum. "Can Involuntary Outpatient Commitment Reduce Hospital Recidivism? Findings From a Randomized Trial with Severely Mentally Ill Individuals." *American Journal of Psychiatry* 156, no. 12 (1999):1968–75. Retrieved from https://www.ncbi.nlm.nih.gov/pubmed /10588412

9. Belluck, P. "Giving Patients a Voice in Their Mental Health Care Before They're Too Ill to Have a Say." *New York Times*, December 3, 2018. Retrieved from https://www.nytimes.com/2018/12/03/health/psychiatric -advanced-directives.html

10. Sample AOT and PAD forms on a hypothetical patient, filled out by Dr. Swartz for the state of North Carolina, can be found at http://www.nrc-pad .org and are also included in the book's resource list on page 197–206.

CHAPTER 6: THE KINDNESS OF STRANGERS

1. *10 Ways Women with Severe Mental Illness Are Overrepresented, Underserved.* Arlington, VA: Treatment Advocacy Center, 2016. Retrieved from https:// www.treatmentadvocacycenter.org/storage/documents/3-26-2019_Women _and_SMI.pdf

2. *Ibid.*

3. Eckert, L. O., N. Sugar, and D. Fine. (2002). "Characteristics of Sexual Assault in Women with a Major Psychiatric Diagnosis." *American Journal of Obstetrics and Gynecology* 186: 1284–91. Cited in *Serious Mental Illness and Homelessness.*

4. *Mass Incarceration: The Whole Pie 2019.* Easthampton, MA: Prison Policy Initiative, 2019. Retrieved from https://www.prisonpolicy.org/reports /pie2019.html

5. Bronson, J., and M. Berzofsky. *Indicators of Mental Health Problems Reported by Prisoners and Jail Inmates, 2011–12.* Washington, DC: U.S.

Department of Justice, Bureau of Justice Statistics, June 2017. Retrieved from https://www.bjs.gov/content/pub/pdf/imhprpji1112.pdf
6. *The 2018 Annual Homeless Assessment Report to Congress.* Washington, DC: Department of Housing and Urban Development, December 2018. Retrieved from https://www.hudexchange.info/resource/5783/2018-ahar-part-1-pit-estimates-of-homelessness-in-the-us/
7. *Ibid.*
8. *Mental Health Courts Program.*Washington, DC: Office of Justice Programs, Bureau of Justice Assistance, n.d. Retrieved from https://www.bja.gov/ProgramDetails.aspx?Program_ID=68
9. Lurigio, A. J. "The First 20 Years of Drug Treatment Courts: A Brief Description of Their History and Impact." *Federal Probation* 72, no. 1 (n.d.).
10. *Mental Health Courts.* Washington, DC: CSG Justice Center, The Council of State Governments, 2019. Retrieved from https://csgjusticecenter.org/mental-health-court-project/
11. Appelbaum, P. S. "Mental Health Courts: A Workaround for a Broken Mental Health System." *Washington Monthly*, June–August 2016. Retrieved from https://washingtonmonthly.com/magazine/junejulyaug-2016/mental-health-courts/
12. Miller, D., and A. Hanson. *Committed: The Battle Over Involuntary Psychiatric Care.* Baltimore, MD: Johns Hopkins University Press, 2016, p. 206.

CHAPTER 7: EARLY AND EFFECTIVE INTERVENTION

1. Saks, E. R. *The Center Cannot Hold: My Journey Through Madness.* New York: Hachette Books, 2008.
2. Marshall, M., S. Lewis, A. Lockwood, R. Drake, P. Jones, and T. Croudace. "Association Between Duration of Untreated Psychosis and Outcome in Cohorts of First-Episode Patients: A Systematic Review." *Archives of General Psychiatry* 62, no. 9 (2005): 975–83. Retrieved from https://www.ncbi.nlm.nih.gov/pubmed/16143729
3. Perkins, D. O., H. Gu, K. Boteva, and J. Liberman. "Relationship Between Duration of Untreated Psychosis and Outcome in First-Episode Schizophrenia: A Critical Review and Meta-Analysis." *American Journal of Psychiatry* 162, no. 10 (2005): 1785–1804. Retrieved from https://www.ncbi.nlm.nih.gov/pubmed/16199825
4. *Ibid.*
5. Andreasen, N. C., D. Liu, S. Ziebell, A. Vora, and B. C. Ho. "Relapse

Duration, Treatment Intensity, and Brain Tissue Loss in Schizophrenia: A Prospective Longitudinal MRI Study." *American Journal of Psychiatry* 170 (2013): 609–15. Retrieved from https://www.ncbi.nlm.nih.gov/pubmed /21059482

6. Annie Wright Psychotherapy. *Neurodiversity: The Next Wave of Mental Health Activism?* November 26, 2017. Retrieved from https://anniewright psychotherapy.com/neurodiversity-next-wave-mental-health-activism/

7. Geoffroy, P. A., and J. Scott. "Prodrome or Risk Syndrome: What's in a Name?" *International Journal of Bipolar Disorder* 5, no. 1 (2017): 7. Retrieved from https://www.ncbi.nlm.nih.gov/pmc/articles/PMC5385319/

8. Norman, R. M. "Are the Effects of Duration of Untreated Psychosis Socially Mediated?" *Canadian Journal of Psychiatry* [*Revue canadienne de psychiatrie*] 59, no. 10 (2014): 518–22.

9. Cannon, T. D., C. Yu, J. Addington, C. E. Bearden, K. S. Cadenhead, B. A. Cornblatt, et al. "An Individualized Risk Calculator for Research in Prodromal Psychosis." *American Journal of Psychiatry* 173, no. 10 (2016): 980–88. Retrieved from https://www.ncbi.nlm.nih.gov/pubmed/27363508

10. *Ibid.*

11. Scharcz, A., and C. E. Bearden. "Early Detection of Psychosis: Recent Updates from Clinical High-Risk Research." *Current Behavioral Neuroscience Reports* 2, no. 2 (2015): 90–101. Retrieved from https://link .springer.com/article/10.1007/s40473-015-0033-6

12. Cannon, T. D., Y. Chung, G. He, D. Sun, A. Jacobson, T. G. M. van Erp, et al. "Progressive Reduction in Cortical Thickness as Psychosis Develops: A Multisite Longitudinal Neuroimaging Study of Youth at Elevated Clinical Risk." *Biological Psychiatry* 77, no. 2 (2015): 147–57. Retrieved from https:// www.sciencedirect.com/science/article/pii/S0006322314004144

13. Sekar, A., A. R. Bialas, H. de Rivera, A. Davis, T. R. Hammond, N. Kamitaki, et al. "Schizophrenia Risk from Complex Variation of Complement Component 4." *Nature* 530, no. 7589 (2016): 177–83. Retrieved from https:// www.ncbi.nlm.nih.gov/pmc/articles/PMC4752392/

14. Owen, M. J., and J. L. Doherty. "What Can We Learn from the High Rates of Schizophrenia in People with 22q11.2 Deletion Syndrome?" *World Psychiatry* 15, no. 1 (2016): 23–25. Retrieved from https://www.ncbi.nlm .nih.gov/pmc/articles/PMC4780289/

15. Brisch, R., A. Saniotis, R. Wolf, H. Bielau, H. G. Berstein, J. Steiner, et al. "The Role of Dopamine in Schizophrenia from a Neurobiological and Evolutionary Perspective: Old-fashioned, but Still in Vogue." *Frontiers in*

Psychiatry 5, no. 47 (2014). Retrieved from https://www.ncbi.nlm.nih.gov
/pmc/articles/PMC4032934/
16. Nutt, A. E. "Suicide Rates Rise Sharply Across the United States, New
Report Shows." *Washington Post*, June 7, 2018. Retrieved from https://www
.washingtonpost.com/news/to-your-health/wp/2018/06/07/u-s-suicide-rates
-rise-sharply-across-the-country-new-report-shows/?utm_term=.
db94b2261320
17. Kowalczyk, L. "Long ER Waits Persist for Children in Mental Health
Crises. *Boston Globe*, July 17, 2018. Retrieved from https://www
.bostonglobe.com/metro/2018/07/17/long-waits-persist-for-children-mental
-health-crises/iD2trxkXIlYtqmsuoqTWII/story.html
18. *Use of Mental Health Services and Treatment Among Children.* Bethesda,
MD: National Institute of Mental Health, n.d. Retrieved January 16, 2015,
from http://www.nimh.nih.gov/health/statistics/prevalence/use-of-mental
-health-services-and-treatment-among-children.shtml

CHAPTER 8: STRENGTH IN (SMALL) NUMBERS, OR AMERICA IS WAKING UP

1. Cloutier, M., M. S.Aigbogun, A. Guerin, R. Nitulescu, A. V.
Ramanakumar, S. A. Kamat, et al. "The Economic Burden of Schizophrenia
in the United States in 2013." *Journal of Clinical Psychiatry* 77, no. 6 (2016):
764–71.
2. Torrey, E. F., R. H. Yolken, and H. R. Lamb. "NIMH Drug Trials for
Schizophrenia." *Journal of Clinical Psychiatry* 80, no. 1 (2019). Retrieved from
https://www.psychiatrist.com/JCP/article/Pages/2019/v80/18com12597.aspx
3. *Global Health Estimates 2016: Disease Burden by Cause, Age, Sex, by
Country and by Region, 2000–2016.* Geneva, SZ: *World Health Organization*,
2018. Retrieved from https://www.who.int/healthinfo/global_burden
_disease/estimates/en/index1.html; Vigo, D., G. Thornicroft, and R. Atun.
"Estimating the True Global Burden of Mental Illness." *The Lancet* 3
(Feburary 2016): 171–78.
4. Kelland, K. "Mental Health Crisis Could Cost the World 16 Trillion by
2030." *Reuters*, October 9, 2018. Retrieved from https://www.reuters.com
/article/us-health-mental-global/mental-health-crisis-could-cost-the-world
-16-trillion-by-2030-idUSKCN1MJ2QN
5. Kessler, R. C., S. Heeringa, M. D. Lakoma, M. Petukhova, A. E. Rupp,
M. Schoenbaum, et al. "The Individual-Level and Societal-Level Effects of
Mental Disorders on Earnings in the United States: Results from the

National Comorbidity Survey Replication." *American Journal of Psychiatry* 165, no. 6 (2008): 703–11.

6. Results from the 2017 National Survey on Drug Use and Health. Rockville, MD: *Substance Abuse and Mental Health Services Administration*, 2018. Retrieved from https://www.samhsa.gov/data/report/2017-nsduh -annual-national-report

7. *National Inpatient Statistics:Outcomes by 659 Schizophrenia and Other Psychotic Disorders.* Agency for Healthcare Research and Quality, Health Cost and Utilization Project, 2013.

8. Taube, C. A., and S. A. Barrett. *Mental Health, United States 1985.* Rockville, MD: National Institute of Mental Health (DHHS/PHS), 1985.

9. Dixon, L. B., and H. H. Goldman. "Medicaid's Institutions for Mental Diseases (IMD) Exclusion Rule: A Policy Debate." *Psychiatric Services*, last modified December 3, 2018. Retrieved from https:// ps.psychiatryonline .org/doi/10.1176/appi.ps.201800412

10. Sisti, D., A. G. Segal, and E. J. Emanuel. (2015). "Improving Long-Term Psychiatric Care: Bring Back the Asylum." *JAMA* 313, no. 3 (2015): 243–44. Retrieved from https://jamanetwork.com/journals/jama/article-abstract /2091312

11. Mathis, M. "Medicaid's Institutions for Mental Diseases (IMD) Exclusion Rule: A Policy Debate." *Psychiatric Services*, 2018. Retrieved from ps.psychiatryonline.org/doi/10.1176/appi.ps.201800413

12. Bond, G. R., R. E. Drake, K. T. Mueser, and E. Latimer. "Assertive Community Treatment for People with Severe Mental Illness: Critical Ingredients and Impact on Patients." *Disease Management and Health Outcomes* 9 (2001): 141–59. Retrieved from https://link.springer.com /article/10.2165/00115677-200109030-00003

13. Han, B., J. Gfroerer, S. J. Kuramoto, M. Ali, A. M. Woodward, and J. Teich. "Medicaid Expansion Under the Affordable Care Act: Potential Changes in Receipt of Mental Health Treatment Among Low-Income Nonelderly Adults With Serious Mental Illness." *American Journal of Public Health* 105, no. 10 (2015): 1982–89; Mark, T. L., L. M. Wier, K. Malone, M. Penne, and A. J. Cowell. "National Estimates of Behavioral Health Conditions and Their Treatment Among Adults Newly Insured Under the ACA." *Psychiatric Services* 66, no. 4 (2015): 426–29. Cited in E. E. McGinty et al., "Communicating About Mental Illness and Violence: Balancing Stigma and Increased Support for Services." *Journal of Health Politics, Policy*

and Law 43, no. 2 (2018): 185–228. Retrieved from https://doi.org/10.1215
/03616878-4303507

14. Dodds, T. J., V. H. Phutane, B. J. Stevens, S. W. Woods, M. J. Sernyak, and V. H. Srihari. (2011). "Who Is Paying the Price? Loss of Health Insurance Coverage Early in Psychosis." *Psychiatric Services* 62 (2011): 878–81. Retrieved from https://www.ncbi.nlm.nih.gov/pmc/articles /PMC4469900/

15. Thomas, K. C., A. Shartzer, N. K. Kurth, and J. P. Hall. "Impact of ACA Health Reforms for People with Mental Hhealth Conditions." *Psychiatric Services* 69 (2018): 231–34. Retrieved from doi:10.1176 /appi.ps.201700044

16. Barry, C. L., H. A. Huskamp, and H. H. Goldman. "A Political History of Federal Mental Health and Addiction Insurance Parity." *Milbank Quarterly* 88, no. 3 (2010): 404–33. Retrieved from doi:10.1111/j.1468-0009.2010.00605

17. Abelson, R. "Mental Health Treatment Denied to Customers by Giant Insurer's Policies, Judge Says." *New York Times*, March 5, 2019. Retrieved from https://www.nytimes.com/2019/03/05/health/unitedhealth-mental -health-parity.html

18. McCance-Katz, E. F. "The Federal Government Ignores the Treatment Needs of Americans With Serious Mental Illness." *Psychiatric Times*, 2016. Retrieved from http://www.psychiatrictimes.com/depression/federal -government-ignores-treatment-needs-americans-serious-mental-illness

19. Rochefort, D. A. (2018). "The Affordable Care Act and the Faltering Revolution in Behavioral Health Care." *International Journal of Health Services* 48, no. 2 (2018): 223–46.

CHAPTER 9: GOING HOME

1. Penn Medicine. *Section II. Institute of the Pennsylvania Hospital Records. Records, Photographic Materials, and Artifacts, 1826–1997.* No date. Retrieved from http://www.uphs.upenn.edu/paharc/collections/finding /iphgeneral.html

2. Appiah, K. A. "May I Cut My Daughter Out of My Life?" *New York Times Sunday Magazine*, The Ethicist, January 8, 2018. Retrieved from https://www.nytimes.com/2019/01/08/magazine/may-i-cut-my-daughter -out-of-my-life.html

3. Lau, M. "In Landmark Move, L.A. County Will Replace Men's Central Jail with Mental Health Hospital for Inmates." *Los Angeles Times*,

February 13, 2019. Retrieved from https://www.latimes.com/local/lanow
/la-me-jail-construction-20190212-story.html

PRACTICAL ADVICE FOR
PERSONS WITH SMI AND THEIR FAMILIES

1. *National Inpatient Statistics: Outcomes by 659 Schizophrenia and Other Psychotic Disorders.* Agency for Healthcare Research and Quality, Health Cost and Utilization Project, 2013.
2. Taube, C. A., and S. A. Barrett. *Mental Health, United States 1985.* Rockville, MD: National Institute of Mental Health (DHHS/PHS), 1985.
3. Amador, X. *I Am Not Sick, I Don't Need Help!* New York: Vida Press, 2012, p. 65.
4. *Ibid.*, pp. 65–66.
5. *Ibid.*, p. 161.
6. Lieberman, J. A., T. S. Stroup, J. P. McEvoy, M. S. Swartz, R. A. Rosenheck, D. O. Perkins, et al. "Clinical Antipsychotic Trials of Intervention Effectiveness (CATIE) Investigators." *New England Journal of Medicine* 353, no. 12 (2005): 1209–23.

INDEX